IMPORTANT NOTE FOR READERS

Encyclopedia of Natural Remedies is an informational guide for a clear and easy understanding of specific illness symptoms and natural ways to treat them if you, your family member, or a friend falls ill. The purpose of this book is not only to read from page to page, but the recipes provided in it deserve to be applied in case of any illness mentioned in it. All the symptoms of every condition are present in this reference manual. Some of the more typical symptoms you might anticipate with this complaint and 'What Causes It?' discuss the likely causes. Sometimes, a complaint is related to what you consume or the environmental conditions; otherwise, it could be caused by inheritance.

You do not need to look further into your illness because you will find here what herbal medicine is. The type of ailment you have with the treatment in the form of herbal remedies and recipes, the limitations and instructions about using these remedies, or safety instructions. So, you can find ways to treat your ailment at home in natural ways in short steps. This book's information should be used as something other than guidance from a qualified healthcare practitioner.

It would help if you got expert medical advice instead of self-diagnosing to treat yourself with natural treatments. Rather, speak with a reputable practitioner, either orthodox or alternative, to get a professional diagnosis.

FROM THE AUTHOR

Hello, I am Paul Dev, an author, blogger, traveler, entrepreneur, horticulturist and alternative medicine practitioner. I run some popular online blogs and published books on various topics. I am extremely enthusiastic and passionate about wellness, health, traveling, business, money, nature etc.

The joy of helping others is one of the biggest things in my life. I have years of expertise in herbal and alternative medicine, so here I am writing this book to help and make people aware of natural remedies backed by science. I hope you will enjoy reading this easy to follow book and find it beneficial.

SCAN & DOWNLOAD OTHER MUST HAVE SUPPORTING RESOURCES

Scan the following QR Code on your phone and download:
- ❏ A 100 Pages Natural Remedies Preparation Planner
- ❏ An Exclusive Herbal Recipes Book
- ❏ A 100 Pages Herbalist journal, and
- ❏ Many more resources will be uploaded gradually that you can download for **FREE**.

Download Now

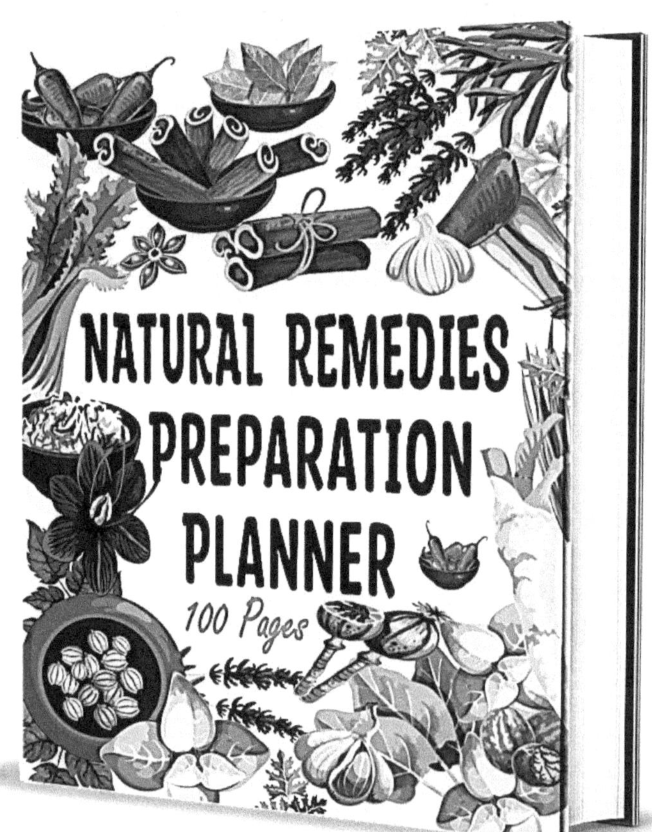

INTRODUCTION

For ages of about 60,000 years, according to archaeological data, people have relied on herbal medicine as a reliable treatment. According to the World Health Organization, 25% of people worldwide utilize herbs for primary healthcare. Up until recently, herbal medicine was the only kind of treatment. Nearly every imaginable treatment was derived from plants since humans began keeping records of their past, perhaps far before.

Ayurveda and Traditional Chinese Medicine are two examples of traditional medical systems that utilize herbal remedies. Indigenous societies (such as African and Native American) also utilized plants in their healing rituals. Researchers discovered that people worldwide frequently used the same or related plants for the same functions.

In the 19th century, the chemicals of plants were being extracted and altered by scientists. That was the time when chemical analysis became possible.

Plants were studied, synthesized, and finally supplanted by medicines, which could produce faster and more potent outcomes as doctors and scientists started to understand the connection between chemistry and disease. Herbal therapies lost favor because most people saw them as quaint and folkloric and relegated to the periphery of modern medicine.

As millions look for a peaceful, natural alternative to traditional care, herbal medicine has reentered over the past few years. Even though many modern medications are now produced synthetically, they were initially derived from plant sources. Herbal medicines use the entire plant, unlike modern conventional medicine, which aims to use only the plant's active component. Depending on whether someone uses inductive reasoning or deductive reasoning to arrive at its utilization, natural medicine first aid may be the first or the final natural remedy they utilize. Herbal medicine is distinct from the traditional medication many of us use.

If you want to treat ingrained issues such as anxiety, high blood pressure, or depression, herbal treatment is more effective. Herbs can be as fast and effective as anything on the drugstore shelf for minor illnesses like colds, cramping, rashes, and skin disorders.

There are two main issues with the use of modern or conventional medicines. The first is the majority of conventional over-the-counter medications for minor health issues are chemically based or contain chemical additives.

The second issue with depending on conventional medicine for minor illnesses is that these treatments mostly reduce symptoms rather than promote healing, if not entirely. Antibacterial spray might prevent an infection from spreading to your cut, but it won't help it heal.

Conventional medicines have some side effects and are not secure to use consistently. For example, the pregnant condition is not allowed to take traditional medicine by healthcare or doctor. In this case, herbal medicines are safe for colds, anxiety, and many more issues. When bacteria adapt to the use of antibiotics, antibiotic resistance develops. Trusted Source resistance grows due to antibiotic abuse and overuse, making it harder to prevent and treat infections. Conventional medicines are expensive and sometimes out of reach. Herbal medicines typically cost less since they are produced from abundant natural materials rather than being synthetically created in a lab. Additionally, they are more straightforward for consumers to access than prescription medications.

Herbal medicine is more suitable in this way. Herbal medicines and remedies are accessible and cost-effective. Herbs are an entirely natural treatment, prevention, and health promotion method. They are a safe and effective alternative or supplement to various pharmacy medications when used as directed and individually recommended for your requirements.

Most specialists concur that herbs can supplement conventional treatments and improve general health because they have distinct but real effects. If you successfully understand the weaknesses and strengths of herbs, you can treat them as medicine more effectively.

Conventional medicines can improve your immunity but with many drawbacks. Since herbal medicine is a natural substance, our bodies can benefit from it. Doctors recommending traditional medicines with years of experience are also starting to hire herbal professionals to treat the diseases more effectively than conventional methods. Doctors and chemists are now starting to mix both treatments (conventional and herbal) to improve the immunity of people.

Always keep in mind that plant medicine is effective and should be taken carefully. We are all unique individuals with unique constitutions and health problems—or lack thereof. Without consulting qualified herbal practitioners and medical professionals, herbal supplements should not be added to pharmaceutical prescriptions already on the patient's prescription list.

TABLE OF CONTENTS

AN INTRODUCTION TO HERBAL MEDICINE & NATURAL REMEDIES

WHAT IS HERBAL MEDICINE?

The use of plants and parts of plants to treat some illnesses is known as herbal treatment. The therapeutic product that is extracted from plants is called herbal medicine. The use of herbs outside of conventional treatment is ancient. Although many modern medications have their roots in plants, they are based on single compounds rather than the numerous active ingredients that plants contain and combine to produce their therapeutic effects. Herbs have a long history of use and can be effective and safe medications when used correctly.

HISTORY AND EVOLUTION OF HERBAL MEDICINE

Herbs and man have a long and devoted history together. Herbs were being used as medicine long before doctors in lab coats began writing prescriptions, even before humans could write. In other words, herbal medicines have been used by humans for the very first time. They are still used by conventional medicine as essential participants in treating many ailments. However, no one can precisely tell the movement when the first person used herbs for healing purposes. Yes, but herbal treatment has been used for thousands of years.

There is an important point to tell the history of herbal medicine. Researchers were researching herbal material history; they found human genetic material on a chunk of yucca herb, which was spit after chewing like a chewing gum ancient form in the American southwest. The age range was from 800-2400 years. Another interesting fact about herbal therapy history is that researchers found the "Ice Man" body that appears to be treated with herbal treatment. That mummy was 3,000 years old and was found in the early 1990s in the Italian Alps. Before the Common Era or formerly BC, researchers discovered chamomile and yarrow that were popular on the teeth plaque of Neanderthals dating back to 60,000 BCE. It showed that humans used plants to treat illness or healing purposes from the beginning before the recorded time.

According to an autopsy, the man had parasitic whipworm infection, leading scientists to surmise that he had probably been administering the medication in regulated amounts to cure them. Herbal medicine developed alongside civilizations throughout the world. And while some of the traditional cures have lost favor, the majority is still widely used today. Imhotep, an Egyptian priest and physician who lived around 2600 S.C. and is frequently credited with penning the first medical writings, provided descriptions of more than 200 ailments' diagnoses and cures, many of which were herbal.

No matter where it is present or originated, every school of herbal medicine is founded on the main idea of herbal treatment. It creates or recreates the state of holistic health and boosts the immunity of the body. Herbalists divide alignments based on symptoms and then use herbal remedies to treat the patients.

Greek civilization, heavily impacted by Egyptian and Middle Eastern cultures, gave rise to Western herbalism. The Greeks employed a system of "humors" connected to the four dynamic elements of air, Earth, water, and fire. The Greeks thought that an imbalance of these humors led to sickness. The humors were a part of each person's personality and weren't always good or evil. But if they lost their equilibrium, illness would follow.

In recent years, scientists have started to work with phytochemicals (chemicals present in plants and responsible for the treatment of disease). They started treating many severe kinds of diseases by using herbal treatment.

There are many remedies scientists have found them to be good for many ailments. Scientists found garlic to be a perfect remedy for stomach health and relaxation. They found that the allicin in garlic is responsible for cholesterol-lowering and antimicrobial activity. 6-gingerol and gingerdione are two compounds that are thought to be suitable for relaxing the stomach.

A compound, capsaicin found in cayenne peppers (*Capsicum annuum, C. frutescens*) reduces pain and acts as a pain killer like conventional medicine but in an effective way and causes heat sensation. The positive thing is that most substances responsible for the repulsion for microorganisms can behave as microbial agents in humans. So, the protective substances for plants can be effective microbial agents for people and can be used for pain reduction, muscle relaxation, and anesthetics.

PLANT COMPONENTS TO TREAT AILMENTS

Most plant secondary components produced for them and used to treat ailments are terpenoids, polyphenols, and alkaloids.

- ❑ *Terpenoids:* Some terpenoids make a plant more appealing to pollinating insects, while others are poisonous or unappealing to grazing animals. Both feverfew (*Tanacetum parthenium*) and chamomile (*Matricaria recutita*) contain terpenoids. Terpenoids are effective for antifungal, anti-inflammatory, immunomodulatory, antihyperglycemic, and antispasmodic effects used to treat and prevent several diseases, including cancer.
- ❑ *Alkaloids:* Alkaloids have strong therapeutic potential. Examples include nicotine, morphine, caffeine, quinine, and nitrogen. Ephedrine is an alkaloid in the Chinese herb ma hang (*Ephedra sinica*). The leaves of the (*Erythroxylum)* coca bush contain cocaine. Cocaine can stimulate the brain and have numbing (anesthetic) effects. The drug cocaine is very addicting. No solid scientific evidence supports using coca leaves for illnesses such as exhaustion, asthma, altitude sickness, and others.
- ❑ *Polyphenols:* Tannins and flavonoids are polyphenol examples. Flavonoids are antioxidant, and it is present in several plants. This class of substances has many more benefits, such as anti-inflammatory activity to treat illness. Tannins is also a beneficial substance used historically to tan animal hides, and they can be found in tea leaves (Camellia sinensis). It is found in grapes (Vitis vinifera) stem, the bark and leaves of bushes and trees such as witch hazel (Hamamelis virginiana).

HOW NATURAL REMEDIES CAN COMPLEMENT CONVENTIONAL MEDICINE

Herbal therapy or medicines have always been used without conventional medicine. The history elaborated on the use of herbal remedies from the very first time when there was no concept of scientific research or traditional way of treatment. Traditional medicine is the term associated with Western method of treatment, including surgery and drugs.

Herbalism is gaining popularity due to its advantages and low rate of side effects. People are proffering herbal treatment over modern therapy. Scientific research also supported plant's phytochemicals' ability to prevent and treat diseases. Plants can improve health by improving immunity. Herbal medicine can be used with conventional medicine in severe conditions. With your doctor's approval, you can also add herbs to many traditional medical treatments.

In many circumstances, the milder characteristics of herbs will serve you much better than the potency that pharmaceutical pharmaceuticals offer. In addition to boosting the effectiveness of conventional medications and/or treatments and counteracting any potential adverse effects, herbs can also be used as adjuncts or complementary therapies. Integrative medicine is a method of treating patients that integrates traditional medicine with CAM practices proven safe and beneficial by science. For instance, ginger (*Zingiber officinale)* can ease nausea brought on by chemotherapy and post-operative procedures.

In other situations, herbs can enhance the advantages of standard medical care. For instance, cancer patients who consume *Cordyceps sinensis* mushrooms after receiving chemotherapy appear to experience increased cellular immunity.

A recent study concluded that Chinese herbs with chemotherapy can stimulate the body's immune system more effectively than chemotherapy alone. Herbs are also used in homeopathy and aromatherapy. These are two other forms of natural healthcare. The practice of applying aromatic plants to treat several diseases and promote general health is known as aromatherapy.

It has its roots in the healing baths and therapeutic massage practices utilized by the ancient Egyptians, Greeks, and Romans. Essential oils are volatile liquids distilled to remove heavy plant waxes, oils, and other components while selecting tiny molecules in modern aromatherapy.

The potency of homeopathic treatments is determined by the process by which the ingredients are diluted and repeatedly shaken (in a procedure known as succussion) until only trace amounts of the original chemical (or none) are left.

WHY DOES HERBAL MEDICINE WORK?

Herbal medicines are used by people to treat or prevent disease. They employ them to relieve symptoms, increase energy, unwind, or reduce weight. The evidence supporting the efficacy of herbal medications is typically relatively scant. While some people find them useful, their use frequently draws more from traditional usage than scientific studies.

Plant growth, soil quality, water quantity, temperature, pests, timing, and method of harvesting are important factors on which the affectivity of the treatment depends. In general, herbal treatment is considered effective compared to conventional treatment.

In addition, unlike medicines that are typically used for an illness, herbs are typically utilized for various conditions. There are some exceptions according to a particular case, but in general, herbal remedies affect the body more than pharmaceutical counterparts.

Most people on Earth use traditional and herbal medicines as their primary form of healthcare. However, complementary and alternative medicine (CAM) use is expanding globally. Up to 80% of people in some nations view herbs as their primary means of remaining healthy.

The fundamental concept of herbalism—and all systems of natural medicine—is that striving for optimal health continuously is preferable to waiting until sickness manifests.

Herbs also have a variety of active ingredients that combine to treat a variety of symptoms as well as underlying issues and improve an organ or system's overall performance. And herbs are frequently combined to promote health.

For instance, licorice (Glycyrrhiza glabra), chamomile (Matricaria recutita), peppermint (Mentha x piperita), and lemon balm (Melissa officinalis) are all included in a multi-herb combination that is used to relieve heartburn, nausea, and vomiting—as well as to support the digestive tract.

And last, it's a rare herb only used to treat one organ or system. Most people treat multiple issues simultaneously, and new evidence supports this all-encompassing strategy. Look for a traditional medicine treatment or pill that can make those claims.

A GENERAL GUIDE TO USING NATURAL REMEDIES

There are several things you should consider when using herbal or natural remedies;

REMEDY ACCESSIBILITY

Wherever you live, you may access most treatments thanks to the increased acceptability of natural therapies. Natural herbs are now sold in towns and cities; you can also order them from online retailers. You should always choose high-quality brands with good-quality herbs that you can afford.

Numerous health food stores and retail businesses that sell products online and consult naturopaths for client advice are available. Apply them! Find out which herbal or supplement blends will work best for you.

WHICH CURE SHOULD YOU PICK?

There will be too many recommended treatments and lifestyle adjustments for you to implement for many conditions. Naturopathic principles recommend starting with the fundamentals. Diet and exercise fit that bill. The best course of action is to eliminate any foods from your diet that are detrimental to your health before considering taking supplements.

Numerous vitamins, minerals, and plants are frequently recommended. Don't be concerned if it doesn't include all of the treatments. Wherever possible, go for a tablet or remedy that naturopaths suggest because these are typically of superior quality and contain the most potent treatments.

DOSAGES

You'll see that I only provided a couple of precise dosages. Dosages have a lot of importance in a remedy. There are some factors to explain about the dosage of herbal treatment:

Everybody is different at all. The body functioning of people is different from each other. Things affect on everybody differently. Some people are more sensitive to drugs, whether they are herbal or synthetic. If a person is sensitive to a 500mg dosage of vitamin C that is too mild, he can have Diarrhea , while others can take a 10,000mg dosage without any adverse effect.

As a measure of protection, it may be an inappropriate dosage if you are not experiencing any benefits from the cure after a reasonable period of time. Asking a qualified professional knowledgeable about the remedy's safety and recommended dosage range is the best line of action.

A note about dose: Side effects are possible with any medication, natural or not.

The exact herbs that are selected are another factor. Any herbalist's education includes learning how to administer dosage. Western herbalists rely on resources of herbs to treat illness. The effectiveness of herbal remedies is influenced by various elements, including growth circumstances, the right time to harvest, the plant parts used, storage, contamination, and freshness.

CHILDREN AND REMEDIES

Although many of the cures are safe for kids, please double-check with your doctor. The dietary suggestions are all suitable for young children.

WHICH DOSE?

The recommended dosage for children is typically stated on the label. However, herbalists' calculations when writing prescriptions for kids are listed below. If you need more clarification, speak with your practitioner.

REACTIONS

The mere fact that a treatment is natural does not guarantee its safety. If you don't feel well or can experience any negative effect, stop using recommended herbs, supplements, and food. Always talk to your trusted practitioner before using treatment. Sometimes, the herbs can also cause reactions. If so, take your time and start with just a little of one thing before going on. It may not work for your body, like with any medication. Fortunately, there are many ways to get to Rome; another treatment option might be more appropriate.

FINAL WORDS

Without any doubt, herbal treatment was the first strategy that the earliest people adopted to treat any illness they faced at that time. With time, herbal treatment started improving by including many different types of therapeutic plants. Scientists are now studying more chemicals present in plants and responsible for treating ailments.

Herbal treatment is using herbs to improve the body system and treat many diseases, including the most dangerous, like cancer. Undoubtedly, herbal treatment can comfort you from pain until you see the doctor. In some cases, this treatment can treat your illness. Herbal treatment can be enough for edema or psoriasis. If you want to find the medical plants for home remedies treatment, it would be quite challenging. The simple thing is to get them from stock pharmacies. A wide variety of herbs is available there. You can also get tinctures, ointments, oils and other products from health food stores that make easy to avoid using conventional medicine.

Health food stores provide herbal treatment variety to make it easy using herbal remedies to treat your illness at home. Gardening of herbs is the other good option when you are living in city or on a farm. You can buy seeds or starter plants at your neighborhood nursery or online. Growing is incredibly satisfying in either case.

Herbs are far safer than prescription medications. But there is something you should keep in mind when using herbal treatments.

Herbal treatment can cause many kinds of reactions depending upon the way of use and dosage of it. The whole herb community considers the extremely rare occurrences of herb-related fatalities to be history. However, errors can occur, and people have died due to overusing and misidentifying toxic herbs. Yes, there are some deadly herbs, although they are not very common. Toxic herbs can cause everything from gastrointestinal irritation to liver and kidney failure. These things are facts, but you can use herbal medicine more safely.

There are more harmful plants in tropical climates. You can take some actions to keep safe. Herbal remedies are treated very differently from pharmaceuticals since they are used in food and supplements compared to conventional ways where drug treatment is standard. Herbal treatment can be some tea, tincture, or balm. There is not any authentic proof of the potency and efficacy of herbal treatment like medical medicine. So, We can't say that all herbal medicines are dangerous; you can use them continuously to stay safe from side effects. Although most herbs pose very little of a danger for interactions or side effects, you should keep an eye on yourself when beginning any new medicine. You must consult a doctor when you start using some herbal treatment. Herbal chemists are also available now to tell you about the chemicals present in the plant you are using and the side effects of it.

Finding a doctor interested in herbs and willing to use them in conjunction with other medical procedures is now very likely. That is the ideal scenario. You must visit a doctor and receive a proper diagnosis if a problem persists for an extended period. Never put off getting checked out; always let your doctor know if you regularly consume any herbs.

If you are elderly, employ caution while using herbal remedies because you may metabolize herbs differently than younger people. The same holds for people who use prescription medicines or have immune system conditions.

Herbs act differently on people with respect to age. Pregnant women have different effects of herbs, and children act differently. Always tell the doctor about your condition and consult about the dosage you use for herbal remedies. So you can stay safe from any reaction and boost your immunity more effectively.

NATURAL REMEDIES FOR 110 MOST COMMON AILMENTS

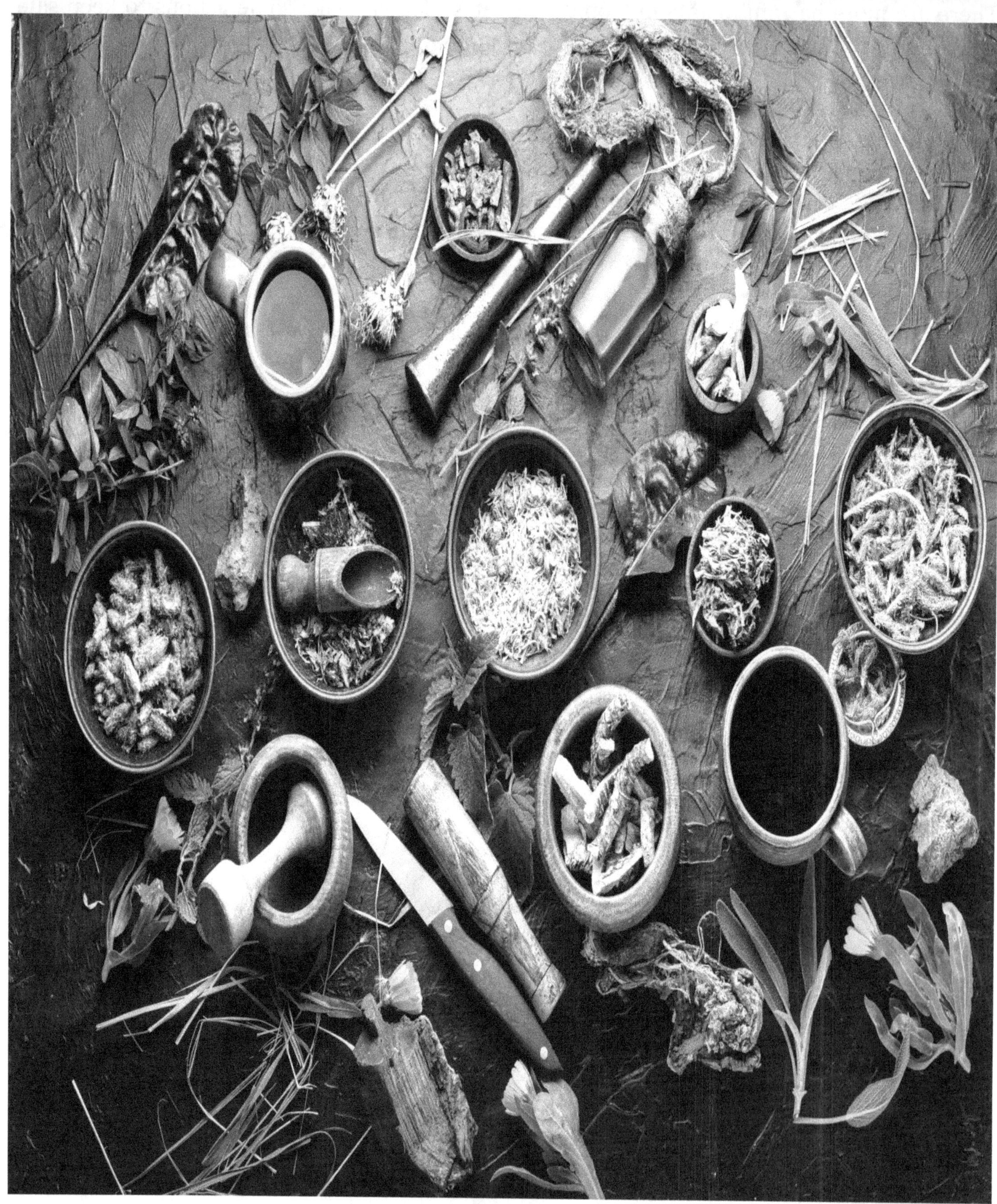

ACNE

Most people face acne when their pores become infected with bacteria or clogged. The common areas where acne mostly breaks out are the face, chest, forehead, upper back, and shoulders. Symptoms of acne include scarring of skin, whiteheads, blackheads, and small red bumps.

NATURAL REMEDIES

1. **Essential Oil :** Take two drops of lavender or tea tree oil and blend with 5 grams of aloe vera gel. Use a cotton swab or clean finger to apply the mixture to blemishes.
2. **Brew Chamomile Tea:** Take a chamomile tea bag and soak it in cold water. If your pimple is inflamed, apply this soaked tea bag directly on your skin for thirty minutes.
3. **Honey and Turmeric:** Honey and turmeric paste are great for acne. Mix an equal ratio of both and make a paste. Apply this directly on the pimple and leave it for 10-12 minutes.
4. **Green Tea Wash:** Prepare a small cup of green tea. Wait until it cools down a little. Use a clean cloth to apply it to the affected area.
5. **Calendula Toner:** Take 2 tbsp of calendula oil and ½ cup of witch hazel. Combine them in a dark glass jar and shake well. Wash your face and apply 5-6 drops on your concern area. Repeat this process twice a day while the acne persists.
6. **Eucalyptus:** Clear your skin with a soothing wash made from grief leaves. Say goodbye to acne-causing bacteria. Alternatively, add essential oils to your morning routine for a fresh start to the day.

Recipes for Treating Acne

Recipe 1: Yogurt Honey Mask
Ingredients:
- 60 g of plain yogurt
- Two strawberries
- 20 g of honey

Instructions:
- Mix strawberries, yogurt, and honey in a small bowl.
- Now clean your face with warm water.
- Apply the mask on your skin with a cotton swab or use a clean, soft brush.
- Wait for 10-15 minutes until fruit and milk acids do their work.
- Use cool water to clean and rinse your face. Pat dry with a clean towel.

Recipe 2: Essential Oil Face Mist
Ingredients:
- 120 ml of witch hazel
- 20 drops of any essential oil
- 115 g of aloe vera gel

Instructions:
- Take a sterilized spray bottle.

- Place the ingredients in the bottle and shake until it mixes well.
- Now, mist this on your face 2-3 times a day.

ALLERGIES

Some people show abnormal immune responses to specific substances. These substances are known as allergens, such as pollens, dust, or even cats' hairs. Allergens are difficult to avoid, as they are present all over our environment, food, and even drinks. **Inflammatory symptoms of allergies include runny nose, swollen eyes, headache, nasal congestion, sneezing, and coughing.**

NATURAL REMEDIES

1. **Ginger:** Take it 2-3 times daily as tincture or tea. Try for a few months to see better results.
2. **Peppermint:**
   - ❏ Mix 3-4 drops of **peppermint oil** and water. Soak a cotton ball into it and chew on it.
   - ❏ While drinking **peppermint tea**, use only natural sweeteners such as honey.
3. **Reishi:** Reishi is best to cure allergies if you take it long-term. You can take it in the form of medical tea or tincture.
4. **Nettles:** If you have nasal allergies, nettles are the best short-term remedy. You can take it in tea or tincture form, which boosts the immune system.
5. **Dried Sage:** Take 235 ml boiling water in a cup and add 2 g of dried sage. Cover and wait for 15 minutes or more. Stain and let it sleep until it cools down to room temperature. Apply this on your skin and let it dry.

<u>Recipes for Treating Allergies</u>

Recipe 1: Salad Dressing to Foil Inflammation
Ingredients:
- 1 tbsp olive oil
- 1 tbsp apple cider vinegar
- 1 tbsp balsamic vinegar
- 1 tbsp flaxseed oil

Instructions:
- Combine the ingredients in a dressing shaker.
- Shake the shaker vigorously ten times to mix the ingredients thoroughly.
- Pour the dressing over your salad.
- Toss the salad to ensure the dressing is evenly distributed.

Recipe 2: Soothing Oat Paste
Ingredients:
- 5 g baking soda
- 5 g colloidal oatmeal
- Add water as needed

Instructions:

- Take a bowl and add colloidal oatmeal and baking soda.
- Stir them together until they blend well.
- Slowly add water as needed to form a paste.
- Apply this paste to the affected area with a clean cotton pad.
- Wait until it dries out, and then wash it off with warm water.

ARTHRITIS

As most people do not know, arthritis is a comprehensive term used to define swelling and inflammation of joints. It commonly elaborates on conditions that distress joints and surrounding tissues. **Its symptoms include pain, stiffness, swelling in joints and restricted motion.**

NATURAL REMEDIES

1. **Turmeric:** Take turmeric and make its paste like curry by adding water. Store this paste in a glass bottle and keep it in the fridge so that it stays longer. Apply this on the affected area to relieve pain 2-3 times daily.
2. **Willow Bark:** Willow Bark can be taken in tea/powdered form or natural pills. Take one dose of natural drugs daily to treat joint pain.
3. **Ginger:** You can make ginger ale and directly sip it or add fresh ginger to your meal. You can also make ginger root tea that relieves stress, tissue, and joint pain.
4. **Comfrey:** It is instructed to use comfrey only externally on pained joints. Never take it internally. You can make oil or salve using comfrey leaves or roots. Use this oil and massage it onto painful joints.

<u>Recipes for Treating Arthritis</u>

Recipe 1: Milding Tea

Ingredients:

- 3 cups of cold water
- 2 tsp of sarsaparilla root
- 3 tsp white willow bark
- 2 tsp yucca herb
- 1 tsp feverfew herb
- 3 tsp of white willow bark

Instructions:

- Take a glass container and combine all the herbs in it.
- Cover the herbs with water and soak them overnight; drain the water and save it in a sterilized glass jar.
- To cure arthritis, take one-half cup 3 times a day.

Recipe 2: Ointment for Arthritis

Ingredients:

- 2 tbsp of chamomile
- 1 pound petroleum jelly
- 2 tbsp of cayenne
- 1 tbsp cayenne

Instructions:

- Take a double boiler and boil petroleum jelly.
- Now add all the mentioned herbs and combine well.
- Heat this mixture for two hours and then remove from heat.
- Take a cheesecloth and pour the mixture through it.
- Before cooling it down, pour warm ointment into the glass jar. Then let it cool down.
- Apply this ointment for arthritis pain and massage it until the skin completely absorbs it.

ASTHMA

This condition of the lungs makes your airways swell and narrow. It also increases the mucus in your body, making your breathing difficult. **Asthma patients face symptoms including shortness of breath, coughing, wheezing, chest pain, and trouble pain.** But remember, every asthma patient has different symptoms.

NATURAL REMEDIES

1. **Coconut Oil:** Try taking a daily coconut oil dose to treat asthma and repair healthy lung tissues. It also counteracts symptoms of asthma. It contains anti-inflammatory properties that increase your ability to absorb nutrients from food.
2. **Apple Cider Vinegar:** Most of us know that combining honey and apple cider vinegar is best for asthma patients. Make a tincture by mixing 1 tbsp of honey and one tbsp of apple cider vinegar in half a cup of lukewarm water. Take it slowly, one sip at a time. You will feel relief over 20-25 minutes, and your breathing becomes easier.

Recipes for Treating Asthma

Recipe 1: Herb Asthma Tea for Quick Results

Ingredients:

- 2 cups of water
- 1 tsp of elecampane root
- 1 tsp of blue vervain leaves
- 2 tsp of horehound herb

Instructions:

- Take all herbs and put them in a pan filled with water.
- First, bring water to the boil and then reduce the heat.
- Leave it to simmer for 25 minutes. After that, strain the water and discard the herbs.
- Wait until the tea cools down. Now asthma tea is ready.

- Take 2 cups of tea daily to treat your asthma.

Recipe 2: Mullein Tea

Ingredients:
- 1 tsp of honey
- 2 tsp of fresh or dried mullein flowers and leaves
- 1½ cups of water

Instructions:
- Use cheesecloth to make a tea bag and place the dried or fresh mullein leaves in it.
- Take boiling water and pour it over the tea bag.
- Now, wait and steep it for 15-20 minutes until it cools down a little.
- Drink it two times a day for any respiratory problems.

Recipe 3: Antioxidant-Rich Waldorf Salad

Ingredients:
- 28 ml of fresh lemon juice
- 75 g of plain Greek yogurt
- 100 g of walnuts
- 150 f chopped celery
- 150 g of sliced seedless red grapes
- Two large peeled, cored, and chopped red sweet apples
- Celery leaves
- ⅛ tsp of each freshly ground black pepper and sea salt
- Pinch of paprika for taste

Instructions:
- Take a large bowl.
- Pour Greek yogurt and lemon juice into it and whip it together.
- Add salt and pepper and stir again.
- Add chopped celery, sliced seedless red grapes, chopped red sweet apples, and walnuts in a separate bowl. Mix them all together.
- Combine yogurt mixture and fruits until fruits are fully covered.
- Add a pinch of paprika to each serving according to your taste.
- Use celery leaves to garnish it.

ATHLETE'S FOOT

Most of us know an athlete's foot with the name of tinea pedis. It is a fungal skin infection. This infection mainly targets those people whose feet become sweaty due to regularly wearing tight-fitting shoes. An athlete's foot is a contagious skin infection that can be spread via clothing, etc. **The symptoms of this infection include continuous itching and scaly rashes.**

NATURAL REMEDIES

1. **Cornstarch:** Cornstarch is the best remedy to treat an athlete's foot at home. You don't need to add anything to it; rub cornstarch on your affected area so it can absorb moisture. If you want to speed up the healing process, add garlic. Garlic is known to kill bacteria. Apply cornstarch at least twice a day to completely disappear fungus.

2. **Vinegar:** If you want to cure your fungal infection (athlete's foot) quickly, vinegar is a must-have thing to try. It burns little, but it is affected. Add vinegar to a tub of water. Use 1:1 to make a soak. Soak your feet into it for 20-30 minutes twice daily for better results. Before putting on your socks or shoes, completely dry your feet.

3. **Garlic:** You can cure your athlete's foot by applying garlic. Mash a clove of garlic with 8 ml of olive oil. Make a fine paste and use it in your affected area. Wash after 60 minutes. But test this remedy on a small skin patch before covering all your feet.

4. **Tea Tree Oil:** Mix 5 ml of tea tree oil with 15 ml of unscented body lotion. Keep blending this mixture in a clean jar. As most of you know, tea tree oil is a powerful natural essential oil, so take precautions while you apply it to the affected area on your feet. When you finish the application process, wash your hands afterwards with water.

<u>Recipe for Treating Athlete's Foot</u>

Recipe: Oregano and Thyme Footbath

Ingredients:

- 5 g of dried thyme leaves
- 6 g of dried oregano
- 946 ml of water
- 72 g of salt

Instructions:

- Take a saucepan full of boiling water to make this relaxing footbath.
- Add all the herbs in water, and cover the saucepan lid.
- Steep the herbs for 20-25 minutes.
- Add salt to the mixture and stir it until salt dissolves.
- Please turn the heat on a low flame and reheat the water until you feel it warm enough.
- Take a basin or tub large enough for your feet and strain water into it.
- Now, soak your feet into this footbath for about 25 minutes.
- Use a clean towel to dry your feet. Make sure to dry your toes.

BACK PAIN

There are different reasons for back pain. The cause can be an accident, sudden weight lifting, or a fall. Back pain develops slowly, but with increasing age, it leads to disability. **Muscle aching, burning sensation, and difficulty in bending or walking are the common symptoms of back pain.**

NATURAL REMEDIES

1. **Chaparral:** This herb contains antioxidant properties. It is known as an excellent herbal remedy for curing back pain. Take chaparral tea 3-4 times a day. This tea cleanses, rebuilds, and tone muscle tissues.
2. **Green Tea:** Drink green tea a minimum of 2 cups daily. It gives you relaxation and also has anti-inflammatory compounds.
3. **Essential Oils:** Different essential oils such as marjoram, chamomile, and lavender oil are the best remedies to try for back pain. These oils contain nervine, sedative, and pain-relieving properties. Take one or more oils and massage your back. You can add them to your bath as needed.

Recipes for Treating Back Pain

Recipe 1: Sciatic Pain Tea

Ingredients:

- 2 cups of water
- 2 tsp of Cramp Bark
- 2 tsp of kava kava root

Instructions:

- Take a saucepan full of water and add all the herbs to it.
- Place the pan on the heat and bring it to a boil.
- After boiling, reduce the heat and simmer for thirty minutes.
- When it cools down, strain the water.
- Drink one cup of this sciatic pain tea per day.

Recipe 2: Soothing Back Pain Tea

Ingredients:

- 2 cups of cold water
- 2 tsp of white willow bark
- 1 tsp of chopped valerian root

Instructions:

- Take a pan and combine all the herbs in it.
- Cover the pan with water and soak overnight.
- Strain and save the water in a clear glass bottle.
- You have to take 1 cup of this daily, one tbsp at a time.

BAD BREATH

Bad breath is interchangeably known as halitosis. If you think that a lack of personal hygiene causes bad breath, you are wrong. It is, but sometimes it happens due to respiratory tract infections and other issues. **Symptoms of bad breath vary from person to person, depending on the underlying cause.**

NATURAL REMEDIES

1. **Baking Soda:** Oral hygiene can be the cause of bad breath. To treat your oral hygiene, brush your teeth with baking soda. Take baking soda and mix it with water to make a thick paste, and use it in place of toothpaste.
2. **Parsley:** Use fresh parsley to treat your bad breath. If you are not comfortable chewing it, make tea with it. But remember, don't add sweetener while making tea, as it would be counterproductive.
3. **Myrrh:** Make a mouthwash to treat your bad breath using myrrh essential oil. Add 3-4 drops of myrrh oil to a cup of warm water. Use this mouthwash daily or as needed.
4. **Peroxide Swish:** Take a clean glass of water and add hydrogen peroxide. Mix well and swish in your mouth for 30-45 minutes. After swishing, spit it out. Rinse your mouth with this twice (morning and evening) a day to cure your bad breath

Recipes for Treating Bad Breath

Recipe 1: Lemon Breath Lift
Ingredients:
- 1 g of stevia
- 235 ml of water
- 28 ml of fresh lemon juice
- 15 ml of pomegranate juice

Instructions:
- Take a glass and pour pomegranate juice and fresh lemon juice into it.
- Add water and stir them all together.
- Now, add stevia into it and combine well.
- Drink this lemon breath lift every morning after your daily routine.

Recipe 2: Mouth Freshening Tea
Ingredients:
- 475 ml of boiled water
- One cinnamon stick
- 2 g of crushed fresh mint leaves
- Two green tea bags

Instructions:
- Add cinnamon sticks, tea bags and mint leaves to the boiling water.
- After one boil, steep for 8-10 minutes. Strain out the herbs and tea bag.
- Drink and enjoy.

BED-WETTING

Nocturnal enuresis or bed-wetting is an **involuntary urination condition.** Before the age of seven, bed wetting wasn't a concern. But after that, if it continues, seek medical help as your child is facing some unstable bladder issues.

NATURAL REMEDIES

1. **Essential Oils:** Use 4-5 drops of any essential oil and put them in the before-bedtime bath. This gives your child relaxation, and he/she feels fresh.
2. **Aspen Essence:** Give your child four drops of aspen essence internally 2-4 times a day. It can help to prevent bed-wetting.
3. **Aloe Vera Juice:** It can be a little uneasy for children to drink aloe vera juice, but it not only stops them from wetting their beds but also makes them less irritable during the night.

Recipe for Treating Bed-Wetting

Recipe: Herbal Tea
Ingredients:
- 1 tbsp of cornsilk
- 1 tbsp of oat straw
- 1 tbsp of horsetail grass

Instructions:
- 2 cups of boiling water
- Take boiling water, add all herbs and steep for about 15-20 minutes.
- Strain and drink this herbal tree 2-3 times a day.

BLACK EYE

Most of us know black eyes with the name of a bruise. It happens when you get a blow to your eye area or forehead that can produce swelling. The cause of the black eye is the broken blood vessels. **Symptoms of the black eye include black and blue bruising, discoloration, and swelling.**

NATURAL REMEDIES

1. **Geranium and Chamomile Oil:** Take 2 tsp of witch hazel and combine it with one drop of chamomile and one drop of geranium oil. Add tbsp of ice-cold water and mix it well. Apply with the help of cotton pads on your closed eyelids and other affected areas.
2. **Prickly Pear Cactus Pad:** Use a prickly pear cactus pad to treat your black eye; it increases the circulation movement in the affected area. Apply the pad to your closed eye and leave it for 20-30 minutes per application. 1-2 applications per day is enough, or you can apply as needed.

BLADDER INFECTION

Cystitis or urinary tract inflammation is called bladder infection. It is the most common type of UTI. Bowel bacteria (like E. coli) are the most common cause of bladder infection. These bacteria reach the bladder through the urethra when the body fails to flush them through urination. **The symptoms of bladder infection include cloudy urine, sudden urges to pee, peeing more frequently, and dealing with pain while peeing.**

NATURAL REMEDIES

1. **Herbal Tea:** Chamomile and ginger teas help soothe bladder discomfort. Drink these teas a few times a day, following package instructions.
2. **Essential Oil:** To fight bladder infections, use special oils. Take a warm bath with Eucalyptus, Juniper, and Thyme oils. Or try Lavender and Sandalwood oils. Use 6–8 drops of each in warm water every day.
3. **Flower Essence :** If you feel overwhelmed with a bladder infection, Flower Essence can help. Patricia Kaminski, who knows about plants and essences, says to use Dill drops. Take four drops four times each day, or more if needed.
4. **Horsetail Herb Tea:** Horsetail herb tea is known for its potential diuretic and anti-inflammatory effects. Drink 1-2 cups of horsetail tea daily, following package instructions.
5. **Vitamin C:** Foods rich in vitamin C, like oranges, strawberries, and bell peppers, can help boost your immune system and create an acidic environment less favorable for bacteria. Include these foods in your daily diet.

Recipes for Treating Bladder Infection

Recipe 1: Cranberry-Apple Drink

Ingredients:

- 1 cup pure, unsweetened cranberry juice
- 1 cup pure apple juice
- One tablespoon fresh lemon juice
- 1-2 tablespoons pure honey (optional)

Instructions:

- Take a glass and mix all their juices.
- Honey is optional if you want to add a more sweet taste.
- Drink the juice 1-2 times daily.

Recipe 2: Herbal Tea Blend

Ingredients:

- One teaspoon dried uva-ursi leaves
- One teaspoon dried dandelion leaves
- One teaspoon dried chamomile flowers
- One teaspoon dried calendula flowers
- 2 cups hot water

Instructions:

- Take a teapot and add all the dried leaves.
- Add hot water to the leaves and leave for 10-15 minutes.
- Strain the leaves and drink the water 2-3 times daily.

BLISTERS

The collection of fluid/serum under the skin is known as a blister. The blisters result in skin damage for various reasons like burns, scratches, allergies, etc. These blisters cause inflammation and hurt. Popping them is not a good idea that leads to spreading infection. **Raised lump filled with clear fluid and reddened patch of skin are clear symptoms of blisters.**

NATURAL REMEDIES

1. **Aloe Vera Gel:** Apply pure aloe vera gel directly to the blister. Use a thin layer several times daily to soothe and speed up healing. Its anti-inflammatory properties will relieve the blisters.
2. **Tea Tree Oil:** Dilute tea tree oil with a carrier oil (like coconut oil) and apply it to the blister. Use a cotton ball to gently dab the mixture on the blister once or twice daily for faster healing and reduced inflammation.
3. **Honey:** Apply a small amount of honey directly to the blister. Cover it with a clean bandage. Change the dressing and reapply honey 2-3 times a day. This will promote healing and minimize inflammation.
4. **Turmeric Paste:** Mix turmeric powder with enough water to create a paste. Apply the paste to the blister and cover it with a bandage. Leave it on for a few hours before rinsing. Use this once a day.
5. **Oatmeal Paste:** Mix oatmeal with water to form a paste. Apply the paste to the blister and leave it on for about 20 minutes. Rinse gently and pat dry. You can do this 2-3 times a day.
6. **Lavender Essential Oil:** Dilute a few drops of lavender oil with a carrier oil and apply it to the blister. Use a cotton ball to gently dab the mixture on the blister once or twice daily.

Recipe for Treating Blister

Recipe: Blisters Soothing Salve

Ingredients:
- 1/4 cup Coconut Oil
- One tablespoon Beeswax Pellets
- 10-15 drops of Lavender Essential Oil

Instructions:
- Melt the beeswax and coconut oil in a boiler and let them cool slightly.
- Add a few drops of lavender oil to the mixture
- Let the mixture solidify again
- Apply the salve on blisters to protect them from infection

BOILS

The bumps developed in internal layers of skin are called boils. **These bumps are usually filled with pus, producing redness and inflammation in the tissues.** The boils form when the skin's normal flora enters hair follicles and causes infection. Usually, boils heal by themselves, but boils cluster/carbuncle can be dangerous if they enter the bloodstream.

NATURAL REMEDIES

1. **Warm Compress:** A warm compress is useful at the initial signs of boiling. Soak a clean cloth in warm water, wring it out, and place it on the boil for about 15 minutes. Apply the warm compress a few times a day to encourage the boil to come to a head and drain.
2. **Tea Tree Oil:** If the boil has drained or opened, apply a small amount of dilute tea tree oil with a carrier oil (such as coconut oil). Use a few drops of tea tree oil mixed with a tsp of carrier oil, applied once or twice daily.
3. **Turmeric Paste:** You can also apply the turmeric paste on an open boil. Apply a thin layer of the paste and leave it on for about 20 minutes, then rinse off. Repeat a few times a day. This will keep the area safe from infection.
4. **Neem Oil:** Neem oil is also best to apply on an open boil. Use a small amount of neem oil and reapply a couple of times a day.
5. **Epsom Salt Bath:** Epsom salt bath is recommended to take throughout the healing process. Add one cup of Epsom salt to a warm bath and soak for about 15-20 minutes. Repeat daily.
6. **Aloe Vera Gel:** Apply pure aloe vera gel to the affected area after the boil has opened and is healing. Apply a thin layer of aloe vera gel several times a day to promote healing and soothe the skin.

BREAST TENDERNESS

Discomfort or pain in the breast, when touched, is called breast tenderness. The degree of tenderness can vary among individuals due to different factors. Medically, this term is known as mastalgia/breast pain. Breast tenderness can be due to pregnancy, hormonal changes, infection, surgery, or any other injury. **Its signs are breast tightness, stabbing pain, aching, and tenderness.**

NATURAL REMEDIES

1. **Cold and Warm Compress:** Apply a warm compress for 15-20 minutes. A warm towel or water bottle wrapped in a cloth can soothe the discomfort and is particularly beneficial before bedtime. On the other hand, a cold compress, like an ice pack wrapped in cloth, can offer immediate relief from acute pain or inflammation.
2. **Flaxseed:** Incorporating flaxseed into your diet can help balance estrogen levels due to its lignan content. You can mix a tablespoon of ground flaxseed into your meals daily.

3. **Evening Primrose Oil:** Primrose oil, containing gamma-linolenic acid (GLA), can regulate hormonal changes that lead to breast pain. Taking 500-1000 mg of evening primrose oil supplements daily, starting a few days before your period and continuing until relief is experienced, can be beneficial.
4. **Vitamin E:** Adequate vitamin E intake through foods like nuts, seeds, and leafy greens can leverage its antioxidant and anti-inflammatory properties to alleviate discomfort.
5. **Dandelion Root Tea:** Dandelion root tea is a natural diuretic, reducing water retention and breast tenderness. Steeping a tsp of dried dandelion root in a cup of hot water for 10-15 minutes and drinking it a few times a week, particularly in the week before your period, can offer relief.

Recipes for Treating Breast Tenderness

Recipe 1: Flaxseed and Berry Smoothie
Ingredients:
- One tablespoon ground flaxseed
- 1 cup mixed berries (strawberries, blueberries, raspberries)
- One banana
- 1 cup almond milk (or any milk of your choice)
- One tablespoon honey (optional for sweetness)
- Ice cubes

Instructions:
- Blend the flaxseed, banana, honey, almond milk, and mixed berries.
- Blend till a smooth cream texture is obtained
- Add ice cubes to blend and crush it. After that, drink it.

Recipe 2: Dandelion Root Tea
Ingredients:
- 1 tsp dried dandelion root
- 1 cup water

Instructions:
- Add dried roots to boiling water.
- Let the roots steep for 10-15 minutes on low flame.
- Stain the roots and enjoy the tea.
- Drink this tea a few times a week.

BRONCHITIS

The inflammation of the bronchial tube is known as bronchitis. Bacterial or viral infection, coughing, irritation, and allergy can cause this inflammation. This inflammation can be acute or long-lasting depending on the cause and immune system. **The major symptoms of bronchitis are fever, sore throat, coughing, shortness of breath, fatigue, discomfort, wheezing, etc.**

NATURAL REMEDIES

1. **Honey and Lemon:** Mix 1-2 tablespoons of honey with freshly squeezed lemon juice in a cup of warm water. Drink this mixture a few times a day. This will provide anti-microbial properties and strengthen your immune system.

2. **Steam Inhalation:** Essential oils like eucalyptus have decongestant properties. Boil water, pour it into a bowl, and add a few drops of essential oils like eucalyptus or tea tree. Lean over the bowl, covering your head and the bowl with a towel, and inhale the steam for about 10 minutes.

3. **Ginger Tea:** Ginger has anti-inflammatory and antibacterial properties, and drinking ginger tea can help soothe irritated airways. Grate a small piece of fresh ginger root and steep it in hot water for 10-15 minutes. You can add honey for taste.

4. **Turmeric Milk:** Turmeric contains curcumin, a compound with anti-inflammatory and antioxidant effects that can help reduce inflammation in the respiratory system. Heat a cup of milk (dairy or plant-based) and add a tsp of turmeric powder. You can also add a pinch of black pepper for better absorption. Drink it before bedtime.

5. **Eucalyptus Oil Chest Rub:** Eucalyptus oil has a cooling effect and can help open up the airways, making it easier to breathe. Mix a few drops of eucalyptus essential oil with a carrier oil (such as coconut oil) and rub it on your chest.

6. **Essential Oil:** Essential oils like eucalyptus, peppermint, or tea tree can be used through methods such as steam inhalation, chest rubs, and diffusion to alleviate congestion and improve breathing.

Recipe for Treating Bronchitis

Recipe: Soothing Herbal Tea

Ingredients:

- 1 tsp of dried thyme leaves
- 1 tsp of dried licorice root
- 1 tsp of dried marshmallow root
- 1 tsp of dried mullein leaves
- 1 tsp of dried ginger root (optional for added warmth)
- Honey (optional, for sweetness)

Instructions:

- Add the thyme, mullein leaves, marshmallow root, licorice root, and ginger root (if using) in 2 cups boiling water.
- Let the herbs steep for 10-15 minutes on low flame.
- Stain the tea and add honey for sweetness (optional)
- Allow the tea to cool slightly before drinking.
- Sip the herbal tea slowly while it's warm. You can drink this tea 2-3 times a day for relief.

BRUISES

A plum-colored area with damaged tissues and ruptured blood vessels is a bruise. A person can get these bruises in case of any injury, surgery, allergy, disease, etc. **By the time the damaged tissues start degrading, resulting in a yellow or green hue, the swelling and tenderness of side tissues also occur.** The human body can deal with minor bruises. However, medications are required to prevent infection and induce faster healing in severe cases.

NATURAL REMEDIES

1. **Cold Compress:** Applying a cold compress to the bruised area immediately after the injury can help constrict blood vessels and minimize swelling. Wrap an ice pack or a bag of frozen vegetables in a cloth and apply it to the bruise for 10-15 minutes. Repeat several times a day.
2. **Arnica Gel or Cream:** Arnica is a natural remedy known for its anti-inflammatory and pain-relieving properties. Applying arnica gel or cream to the bruise can help reduce swelling and alleviate discomfort. Follow the product instructions and avoid using broken skin.
3. **Pineapple or Papaya:** These fruits contain enzymes (bromelain in pineapple and papain in papaya) that may help reduce inflammation and improve circulation. Consuming fresh pineapple or papaya or applying them as pulp to the bruise might aid healing.
4. **Witch Hazel:** Witch hazel has astringent properties that can help shrink blood vessels and reduce swelling. Soak a cotton ball in witch hazel and gently dab it on the bruised area a few times daily.
5. **Turmeric Paste:** Turmeric contains curcumin, which is known for its anti-inflammatory properties. You can apply the turmeric paste with water or aloe vera gel to cover the wound for 15-30 minutes.
6. **Elevation:** Elevating the bruised area can help reduce blood flow and minimize swelling. This is particularly effective for bruises on the limbs.

Recipe for Treating Bruises

Recipe: Pineapple and Papaya Bruise Soothing Smoothie
Ingredients:
- 1 cup fresh pineapple chunks
- 1/2 cup fresh papaya chunks
- One banana
- 1/2 cup coconut water or water
- Ice cubes (optional)

Instructions:
- Add all the fruits in a blender with coconut water.
- Blend the fruits until a smooth, creamy smoothie is ready. Add ice if required.
- Consume the smoothie once a day.

BURNS

Tissue injury that is caused due to the exposure of chemicals, radiation, fire, or electricity is known as burn. Based on the cause and damage severity, these burns are divided into 3 major types. **Burns cause blisters, inflammation, redness, pain, peeling of skin etc.**

NATURAL REMEDIES

1. **Cool Water:** Hold the burn under cool running water for 10-15 minutes immediately after the injury. This helps to cool the skin, reduce pain, and prevent further damage.
2. **Aloe Vera Gel:** Apply a thin layer of pure aloe vera gel to the burned area. Aloe vera has anti-inflammatory and soothing properties that can help relieve pain and promote healing.
3. **Honey:** Honey has natural antibacterial properties and can create a protective barrier over the burn. Apply a thin layer of raw, organic honey to the burn and cover it with a sterile dressing.
4. **Lavender Essential Oil:** Dilute a few drops of lavender essential oil in a carrier oil (such as coconut or olive oil) and gently apply it to the burn. Lavender oil has soothing and healing properties that can aid in burn recovery.
5. **Potato Slices:** Cut a raw potato into thin slices and place them directly onto the burn. Potatoes have cooling and anti-irritant properties that can provide relief.
6. **Calendula Tincture:** Calendula (marigold) flowers have natural wound-healing and anti-inflammatory properties. Calendula tincture can be used to disinfect and soothe the burn area. Apply the diluted tincture to the burn using a clean cotton ball or swab. Let it air dry. If needed, you can also apply a clean, sterile bandage over the burn. Repeat this process a few times a day.

Recipe for Treating Burns

Recipe: Honey and Coconut Oil Burn Treatment

Ingredients:
- Raw, organic honey
- Virgin coconut oil
- Clean, soft cloth or sterile gauze
- Cold water

Instructions:
- Gently rinse the burn area with cold water to clean it.
- Mix equal amounts of virgin coconut oil and honey in a small bowl and make a smooth mixture.
- Apply a thin layer of mixture on the burn with clean hands.
- If needed, cover the treated burn with a clean, soft cloth or sterile gauze to protect it from outside contaminants.

CANKER SORES

Canker sores are interchangeably known as aphthous ulcers. They look like small and shallow lesions that mostly occur in the soft tissues of your mouth. They also develop in base gums, which makes your eating and talking difficult. **Burning sensations and tingling are the common symptoms of canker sores.** Most of them are round or in oval shape with blood-red borders. Seek medical attention if canker sores are large or painful and don't go away alone in a week or two.

NATURAL REMEDIES

1. **Licorice Tea:** Licorice tea is used to heal canker sores as it gives a soothing feeling to your mouth. Take 1-2 big cups slowly of this herbal tea per day. Make sure to retain the tea in your mouth for a few seconds before swallowing.
2. **Yarrow Special Formula:** Yarrow is known as a fundamental healing agent. It is best to treat canker sore as it strengthens your body against stress and bacteria. To treat canker sore, take four drops of yarrow formula per day or according to your need.

Recipe for Treating Canker Sore

Recipe: Essential Oil Blend

Ingredients:

- Five drops of lemon
- Ten drops of eucalyptus
- 5 drops of helichrysum
- Five drops of geranium
- Ten drops of lavender
- Five drops of bergamot

Instructions:

- Take a jar and add all these essential oils.
- Add ½ ounce of vegetable glycerin.
- Use a clean finger or cotton swab for the application of this blend.
- Apply this blend on your canker sore 3-4 times daily.

CARPAL TUNNEL SYNDROME

Carpal tunnel syndrome (CTS) is one of the most common hand conditions in which a person feels a tingling sensation in his hand. In most cases, this condition persists for months and even gets worse with time. The main cause of carpal tunnel syndrome is when a nerve in your wrist is pinched due to usual day-to-day activity. **Feeling numbness and tingling in your hands are the common symptoms of CTS.** Comparing to men, women are 3 times more like suffer from carpal tunnel syndrome. It can happen to anyone but normally it occurs in adults mostly. Lifestyle factors like smoking, high body mass index (BMI), high salt intake etc. increase the risk for this.

NATURAL REMEDIES

1. **Ice Therapy:** Using ice packs is good for numbing the pain of carpal tunnel syndrome. Take ice packs, cover them with a towel, and wrap them around the waist joint. Remove it after 20-25 minutes. You can also use an ice bath to treat CTS. Take a bowl full of water and ice. Soak your hand into it for 10-15 minutes.
2. **Stay Warm:** Carpal tunnel syndrome becomes worse if you don't pay attention. Make sure to keep your hands warm.

CHRONIC PAIN

If you are facing any pain for as long as three months and no medication is affected, you have chronic pain. There are many causes of chronic pain, including arthritis, other injury, or any other elusive case. **The symptoms include severe pain, insomnia, aching, anxiety, burning, and tiredness.**

NATURAL REMEDIES

1. **Fish Oil:** Taking 1200 milligrams of fish oil per day can treat your chronic pain.
2. **Resveratrol:** Taking resveratrol can help you as it works on a cellular level for pain regulation. It has very beneficial effects, such as anti-cancer or even life-prolonging benefits.
3. **Turmeric:** People with chronic pain can have turmeric with two other substances, bromelain and devil's claw, as it gives noticeable pain relief.

COLD SORES

The cause of cold sores is a virus, HSV, which makes them contagious. These sores are usually formed around the lips and are filled with fluid. **This condition causes fever, burning/itching/tingling around the mouth, inflamed glands, nausea, pain etc.** A person with a weak immune system can develop these sores more frequently. The sores last 7-10 days in general.

NATURAL REMEDIES

1. **Ice:** Applying ice wrapped in a cloth directly on the cold sore for 15 minutes every hour can help reduce pain and swelling. This can be especially effective during the early stages when you feel the tingling sensation that precedes the outbreak.
2. **Lip Balm with Sunscreen:** Regularly applying lip balm with sunscreen can shield your lips from further sun exposure. It can trigger or worsen cold sores. Keeping your lips moisturized can also prevent cracking and discomfort.
3. **Aloe Vera Gel:** Apply a thin layer several times daily to help speed up the healing process and provide relief.
4. **Tea Bags:** Applying a warm, damp tea bag to the cold sore for 15-20 minutes a few times daily can help soothe and promote healing.

5. **Lysine Supplement:** Taking lysine supplements as directed can help prevent outbreaks and reduce the frequency of cold sores. Always consult a healthcare professional before starting any supplements.

Recipes for Treating Cold Sore

Recipe 1: Tea Tree Oil and Coconut Oil Cold Sore Treatment

Ingredients:
- 2-3 drops of tea tree essential oil
- One teaspoon of virgin coconut oil
- Clean cotton swab or Q-tip

Instructions:
- Mix a tea tree and coconut oil in a small container.
- Apply the mixture on the sores with clean cotton swabs gently. Avoid using fingers to prevent cross-contamination.
- Apply the mixture 2-3 times daily or as needed for relief. Make sure to use a fresh cotton swab each time.

Recipe 2: Herbal Compress

Ingredients:
- 1 cup dried calendula flower, plantain leaf, chamomile flower, linden leaf and flower each
- ½ cup dried St. John's wort leaf and flower
- ½ cup dried self-heal leaf and flower

Instructions:
- Mix well with the dried leaves and flowers in a large bowl. Store them in an airtight container.
- Mix 2-3 tablespoons of herbal mixture in boiling water. Put the herbal medicine into a mason jar/French press. Pour the boiling water over the herbs, cover the jar or press, and steep for about 20 minutes. During this time, you can also prepare a hot water bottle.
- Dip the cloth in a warm herbal infusion, gripping it by a dry corner, and let it slightly cool until it becomes warm to the touch, ensuring it's comfortably hot.
- Gently press the cloth on the affected area for 10-20 minutes. Repeat the process 2-3 times a day.

COLIC

Excessive, prolonged, intense crying or fussiness in newborn babies for no obvious reason is known as colic. It's not a disease but a medical term. It is estimated that 5% to 28% infants experience this during their first few months of lives. **The symptoms include excessive crying and gas, clenched fists, hard to calm the baby, red face, and bringing knees to chest.** This condition can last about 3 days a week or three hours a day. Colic is not harmful but can cause discomfort for both baby and parents. Difficulty in digestion, burping, insensitivity, and over/underfeeding can be a few causes of colic.

NATURAL REMEDIES

1. **Swaddling:** Swaddling your baby snugly in a blanket can provide security and comfort. It may also help prevent your baby's arms from flailing, which can reduce fussiness.
2. **Gentle Massage:** Massaging your baby's tummy clockwise can help alleviate gas and digestive discomfort. Use baby-safe oil, and be sure to apply gentle pressure.
3. **Bicycle Legs:** Lay your baby on their back and gently move their legs in a cycling motion. This can help relieve gas by promoting movement in the digestive system.
4. **Probiotics:** Consult your pediatrician about using infant-friendly probiotics. These can help balance the gut bacteria and potentially reduce colic symptoms.
5. **White Noise or Soft Music:** Soft, calming sounds like white noise or gentle music can help distract and soothe a fussy baby. There are various white noise machines or apps designed specifically for infants.
6. **Chamomile Tea (for breastfeeding mothers):** Drinking chamomile tea might help soothe your baby's digestive system if you are breastfeeding. The soothing properties of chamomile can be transferred through breast milk. However, always consult your doctor before trying this.
7. **Carry and Comfort:** Holding your baby close in a baby carrier or sling can provide comfort through the warmth of your body and the rhythmic motion of your movements. Many babies find this soothing.

Recipe for Treating Colic

Recipe: Digestive Massage Oil

Ingredients:

- 1 tbsp carrier oil (such as coconut oil or olive oil)
- 1 drop of high-quality, infant-safe peppermint essential oil (optional)
- 1 drop of high-quality, infant-safe lavender essential oil (optional)

Instructions:

- Mix all the oils in a small bowl. Make sure that the essential oil you are using is safe for infants.
- Test the mixture on your skin for irritation or reaction.
- Gently massage the oil on the baby's tummy in a clockwise direction.
- Repeat the process daily if you notice any comfort in the baby after the massage.

COMMON COLD

The common cold is the contagious upper respiratory infection of the airways caused by viruses. There are more than 200 viruses that can cause colds. **The most significant cold symptoms are runny nose, sore throat, throat pain, coughing, sneezing, and scratchy throat.** Most of the time common cold is harmless. Normally a cold may last for around a week, whereas few colds last longer. Children, aged and adults those are in poor health suffer prolonged colds. Typically, a person can catch 2-4 colds/year, while the kids might get double it.

1. **Honey:** Honey can help soothe a sore throat and cough. Never give honey to infants under one year old due to the risk of botulism. Adults can take 11-2 tsp of raw honey three times daily. For children over 1 year old, half to 1 tsp is enough.

2. **Steam Inhalation:** Add a few drops of eucalyptus or peppermint essential oil to a bowl of hot water. Lean over the bowl, cover your head with a towel, and inhale the steam. Take the steam 2-3 times a day. It helps relieve nasal congestion, soothing irritated throat, and loosening mucus, providing comfort and temporary relief.

3. **Salt Water Gargle:** Mix 1/4 to 1/2 teaspoon of salt in a cup of warm water. Gargle every few hours as needed. Gargling with salt water can help soothe a sore throat. Make sure to avoid swallowing the solution.

4. **Ginger Tea:** Use one teaspoon of freshly grated ginger or 1/2 teaspoon of dried ginger per cup of water. Take 2 to 3 cups a day. Steep ginger in hot water for 10 minutes, strain, and add honey and lemon if desired.

Recipe for Treating Common Cold

Recipe: Super Elderberry Syrup
Ingredients:
- 1 cup dry elderberries
- 2 tbsp dry echinacea root
- Dry astragalus root 3-4 slice
- 1 tsp dry clove
- 2 inches fresh ginger piece
- One cinnamon stick
- 4 cup water
- 1 cup fresh raw honey

Instructions:
- Add all the ingredients and water to a large pot except honey and boil them.
- When the water starts boiling, leave them for 45 minutes on low flame.
- After the water remains half, let the mixture cool.
- Strain the mixture with the help of a thin, clean cloth and let it cool completely.
- Add the honey to the cold mixture and mix well. You can store the syrup for about one year and use it.

CONJUNCTIVITIS

Conjunctivitis is an eye condition or inflammation that caused by infection or allergies. Conjunctivitis, also known as pink eye, is a contagious disease It is the swelling of the conjunctiva, the thin mucous member inside the eyelid. It's also called pink eye because the white part of the eye turns pink or red in this condition. Bacteria and viruses can both be the cause of this condition. **The common symptoms are red eyes, irritation, swelling, and excessive tear production.**

NATURAL REMEDIES

1. **Chamomile Tea:** Take a tea bag of plain chamomile tea and place it into a hot water cup for about 2 minutes. Remove the tea bag and let it cool completely. Close the infected eye and press the tea bag for 10-20 minutes.
2. **Castor Oil Compress:** You can briefly apply a small amount of castor oil to a sterile cotton ball and place it on your closed eyelids. Be cautious not to get the oil directly into your eyes.
3. **Witch Hazel:** You can soak a cotton ball in witch hazel to reduce irritation and gently dab it around the eyes.
4. **Rose Water:** With the help of a sterile dropper, you can place a few drops of pure rose water into each eye. Ensure you use high quality rose water that contains no additives.
5. **Cold Compress:** You can take a slice of chilled potato or cucumber and place it on closed eyes for a few minutes. Repeat the process when you feel the discomfort again.

Recipe for Treating Conjunctivitis

Recipe: Warm Milk and Honey Compress

Ingredients:

- 1/4 cup of milk
- One teaspoon of honey
- Clean, soft cloth

Instructions:

- The milk should be heated in the microwave or on the hob until it is warm enough to drink.
- Once the honey is added, thoroughly mix it in.
- In the heated milk and honey mixture, dunk a clean towel.
- Gently squeeze the extra liquid out of the cloth.
- The heated towel should be placed over your closed eyelids.
- For ten to fifteen minutes, leave the compress in place.
- After removing the compress, gently rinse your eyes with cool, fresh water.

CONSTIPATION

The difficulty in releasing the stool due to hardness, infrequent stool, and less bowel movement refers to constipation. It is estimated that more than 4 million people in the United States have frequent constipation. The primary reason for constipation is low fluid and fiber intake. While certain medications ignore the urge to pee, less physical activity and other things can cause constipation. It's signs are:

- **Difficulty and pain in passing stool**
- **Less frequent bowel movement**
- **The feeling of rectum blockage and irritation**

Constipation is fairly common and people of all ages experience constipation from time to time.

1. **Psyllium Husk:** Husk turns into a jelly-like substance in liquid, it becomes easier to pass the stool after its intake. Mix ½ cup of water into ½ cup of apple juice, add two tsp of psyllium husk, and stir well. Drink this 2-3 times a day.
2. **Flaxseeds or Chia Seeds:** These seeds are high in soluble and insoluble fiber, which can aid in softening stools and promoting regularity. Add them to yogurt, smoothies, or oatmeal.
3. **Prune Juice or Prunes:** Consume a small glass of juice in the morning on an empty stomach. If you want to eat, have 3-4 prunes daily; otherwise, excessive intake can cause extreme bloating or gas.
4. **Flaxseeds and Psyllium Smoothie:** Blend the 1½ flaxseed meal with half a banana, a few strawberries/raspberries, 1 tsp psyllium, and almond milk. Add ice if required. Blend till a smooth mixture is prepared, and enjoy. You can have this smoothie once a day.

<u>Recipe for Treating Constipation</u>

Recipe: Brocco-licious Fiber-Rich Salad

Ingredients:

- 2 cups fresh broccoli florets, steamed or blanched
- 1 cup cooked quinoa
- 1/2 cup cooked black beans
- 1/4 cup chopped prunes (dried plums)
- 1/4 cup chopped almonds or walnuts
- One tablespoon olive oil
- One tablespoon lemon juice
- One teaspoon honey or maple syrup (optional)
- Salt and pepper to taste

Instructions:

- Steam broccoli until tender-crisp; set aside.
- Cook quinoa as directed; fluff with a fork.
- Mix broccoli, quinoa, beans, prunes, and nuts.
- Add oil, lemon juice, honey, salt, and pepper to the salad.
- Drizzle dressing over the mixture; gently toss.
- Serve and savor this fiber-rich salad.

COUGH

Coughing is a protective reflex that the body cleans the lungs and airways. It is the body's defence against foreign particles entering the airways. When particles like viruses, smoke, particles, and pollens enter the body with air, this mechanism stops them before they reach the lungs. Viruses are the most common agent. **The signs of coughing include airway tissue damage, sleep problems, vomiting, hoarseness, runny nose, and sore throat.**

NATURAL REMEDIES

1. **Honey:** Consume 1 to 2 teaspoons of raw honey directly or mix it with warm water or herbal tea. The kids of >1 year can take ½ tps but avoid giving it to infants. You can also use 1 tsp of honey with peppermint essential oil 3-4 times a day. Mix 4-5 drops of oil with 1/4 cup of honey and put in a jar to use all day.
2. **Peppermint Tea:** Peppermint tea with the addition of thyme gives a calming effect against cough. Add 3 tsp of dry peppermint leaves and 1 tsp of thyme leaves in 2 cups boiling water - steep the leaves in water for 15 minutes and strain. Drink tea a few times a day.
3. **Steam Inhalation:** Inhale steam from a bowl of hot water. Add eucalyptus or peppermint essential oil if desired. Perform steam inhalation for 10-15 minutes, 2 to 3 times a day.
4. **Essential Oils:** Inhale the lavender which will help improve the blood flow and reduce inflammation.
5. **Rosemary inhalation:** Add ½ cup of dried leaves in boiling water. Let the leaves soak thoroughly and inhale the steam for 10-15 minutes.

Recipes for Treating Cough

Recipe 1: Honey Lemon Ginger Tea

Ingredients:
- One tablespoon honey
- One tablespoon freshly squeezed lemon juice
- One teaspoon grated fresh ginger
- 1 cup hot water

Instructions:
- Add all the ingredients to a cup and pour boiling water.
- Leave the water for a few minutes, and add honey if required.
- Slowly drink the tea to soothe the throat from pain and irritation.

Recipe 2: Honey and Cinnamon Cough Syrup

Ingredients:
- Two tablespoons honey
- 1/2 teaspoon cinnamon powder

Instructions:
- Mix honey and cinnamon powder in a small bowl.
- Take a teaspoon of this mixture as needed to soothe cough and irritation in the throat.
- Swallow the mixture slowly, allowing it to coat your throat for relief.

CUTS AND SCRAPES

These small wounds damage our skin and sometimes open the internal tissue layers unlike scrapes that usually affect the upper layers. Cuts can harm the deeper tissues and blood vessels. **Cuts and scratches cause swelling, pain, irritation, and bleeding.**

NATURAL REMEDIES

1. **Aloe Vera Gel:** Extract the gel from the leaf and apply it to the wound with a clean finger. You can also mix the gel with honey or turmeric to enhance its effect.
2. **Chamomile Tea Compress:** Make chamomile tea by adding the dry leaves in boiling water. Leave the water for 15 minutes and let it cool. Soak a clean cloth in it. Apply the cloth as a compress to the wound.
3. **Coconut Oil:** Apply a thin coconut oil layer to moisten the wound and promote healing.
4. **Turmeric Paste:** Make a paste using turmeric powder and water, and apply it to the wound.
5. **Witch Hazel:** Apply witch hazel, a natural astringent, to help cleanse and soothe the wound. It can also reduce inflammation.
6. **Tea Tree Oil:** Dilute tea tree oil with a carrier oil and apply a small amount to the wound.

Recipe for Treating Cuts and Scrapes

Recipe: Homemade First-Aid Salve

Ingredients:

- 1/4 cup olive oil or coconut oil (or a combination of both)
- Two tablespoons beeswax pellets or grated beeswax
- 10-15 drops of tea tree essential oil
- 10-15 drops of lavender essential oil
- *Optional:* 5-10 drops of vitamin E oil

Instructions:

- Take a large pot with boiling water and place a heat-resistant bowl in water. Add the olive oil/coconut oil to a bowl.
- Let the oil melt completely on medium flame.
- Add beeswax pellets into the oil and let melt by stirring.
- Once the oil and beeswax are combined, remove the bowl from the heat and let it cool slightly.
- Add a few drops of essential oil to the mixture and mix well.
- Place the mixture in a clean jar and let it dry.
- Apply the salve on the wound with a clean finger a few times a day.

DANDRUFF

Dandruff is a skin condition caused by fungal infection. In this condition, the skin on the scalp starts to flake and is unpleasantly itchy. Dandruff is not dangerous, but it can be embarrassing. **Various signs show you are dealing with dandruff, such as itchy, scaly, and crusty scalp.**

NATURAL REMEDIES

1. **Apple Cider Vinegar:** To treat dandruff:
   - Use an old shampoo bottle and fill it with apple cider vinegar.
   - Before the bath, apply this apple cider vinegar to your scalp and hair.

- ❑ Gently and deeply rub it in and leave it for half an hour.
- ❑ Then wash your hair.

2. **Lemon Juice and Aloe Vera:** Take one tsp of gel of aloe vera and combine it with lemon juice. Rub this mixture into your scalp. Leave it for 2-3 minutes. Then wash your hair with fresh water.
3. **Coconut Oil:** Massage your hair and scalp with virgin coconut oil. Wait for 20 minutes, and then shampoo your hair.
4. **Tea Tree Oil:** Combine a few drops of tea tree oil with coconut oil or shampoo. Apply to your scalp and leave it for a few minutes. Then shampoo as usual.
5. **Baking Soda:** Take a tbsp of baking soda and sprinkle it onto your scalp. Wait for 1-2 minutes and wash your hair.
6. **Green Tea:** Add green tea to the apple cider vinegar. And combine well. Sprinkle it on your scalp and allow it to sit for about 3-5 minutes. Then, shampoo your hair.

Recipe for Treating Dandruff

Recipe: Rosemary Scalp Wash

Ingredients:
- 235 ml of apple cider vinegar
- 3 g of fresh rosemary leaves

Instructions:
- Take a small pan and pour vinegar into it.
- Heat it until it starts boiling.
- Turn off the heat. Add fresh rosemary leaves and stir them.
- Cover the pan and wait for 10-15 minutes.
- Discard herbs and save the mixture in a clean, empty bottle.
- Rinse your scalp with 60 ml of prepared solution and 475 ml of water.

DEPRESSION

Depression is a behavioural disorder in which your mood swings. In most cases, you feel constant sadness and lose interest even in your daily tasks. It causes a variety of emotional and physical issues. **Daily episodes of depression may include tearfulness, hopelessness, loss of pleasure, sleep disturbance, lack of energy, etc.** Depression is a very common mental health condition. Worldwide 5% adults suffer from depression.

NATURAL REMEDIES

1. **Apple Cider Vinegar:** Take 1 tsp of apple cider vinegar daily to treat depression. It works as a liver-cleaning tonic and helps with serotonin levels in the brain.
2. **Scatter Joy:** You can treat your depression only by yourself. Try to smile more often at someone who could be your family, friend, or animal. Try to talk with people around you, say hello, and learn about them.

3. **Flower Essences:** Pine essence is best for those depressed, accompanied by regret and loss. Borage is for those who are dealing with depression accompanied by grief.
4. **St. John's Wort Herb:** Try taking 300mg of St. John's Wort herb. After a few weeks, you will feel relaxed.
5. **Lemon Balm:** For treatment, you can take lemon balm as tea or tincture. It can help with mild depression, and you will feel the effects after some time.

Recipe for Treating Depression

Recipe: Antidepressant Tea

Ingredients:
- 1 tbsp of lemon balm leaf
- 1 tbsp of hawthorn leaf or berry
- 2 tbsp of St. John's wort leaf or flower
- Eight oz. of hot water

Instructions:
- Take a pan and combine all herbs in water.
- Covered and stepped for about 15-20 minutes.
- Discard the herbs and take tea slowly.
- You can add honey to your tea to sweeten it according to your taste.

DIABETES

This condition includes type 1 and 2 diabetes. Chronic diabetes happens when your body's blood sugar level increases more than usual. The symptoms of diabetes vary and depend on how much your blood sugar level is high. **Some symptoms include urinating often, feeling weak and tired, mood swings, thirstiness, losing weight, and many more.**

NATURAL REMEDIES

1. **Jamun Seeds:** Take dehydrated 20-25 jamun seeds in powdered form and consume 2 tbsp daily. Jamun seed is best for treating diabetes as it stimulates insulin production and reduces the glycemic load.
2. **Curry Leaves:** Make a tea of curry leaves with cinnamon and a little ginger. Take this tea twice a day. Curry leaves offer various benefits, like aiding digestion, regulating blood sugar levels, and improving insulin sensitivity.

Recipe for Treating Diabetes

Recipe: Roasted Veggie Explosion

Ingredients:
- 15-30 ml of olive oil
- One large onion
- 7 g of crushed fresh rosemary
- Sea salt, according to taste

- One yellow bell pepper (sliced into strips)
- One bunch of woody bottoms cuts asparagus
- Two peels and quartered beets
- Two peeled garlic cloves

Instructions:
- Preheat your oven to 200 centigrade.
- Spray olive oil on your baking sheet.
- Take your vegetables in a large bowl and drizzle some olive on them. Combine them well until they all are fully coated with olive oil.
- Spread garlic and all other vegetables on your baking sheet, and sprinkle some sea salt and fresh rosemary to give it a flavor and aroma.
- Put this tray in a preheated oven and wait 15 minutes until they are roasted. Flip the vegetables and roast for another 10 minutes.
- They are ready to eat when golden brown and have crispy edges.

DIAPER RASH

Diaper rash is also known as dermatitis. The most common causes of diaper rashes are wet diapers, the infrequency of changing diapers, chafing, and skin sensitivity. **The most common signs of diaper rashes are sores on your baby's bottom, crying, itching, and inflamed skin.**

NATURAL REMEDIES

1. **Apple Cider Vinegar:** Mix 1:1 water and apple cider vinegar. Apply this solution with a wet cotton swab on the baby's skin before each diaper change. Mix it with freshly brewed and cold red bush tea in the same ratio. Both of these remedies are known as effective cures for various rashes.
2. **Chamomile and Echinacea Gel:** Mix chamomile and echinacea with aloe vera to make a gel. This gel is perfect to heal and soothe your baby's rash. You can make this gel and store it in the refrigerator.
3. **Calendula Caress Flower Oil:** This flower oil eases the baby's diaper rash and is soothing. Apply this calendula caress flower oil whenever you change your baby's diaper.
4. **Aloe Vera Gel:** Apply aloe vera gel topically every time you change the baby's diaper. This gel is famous for its skin-healing properties.

Recipes for Treating Diaper Rash

Recipe 1: Comforting Diaper Cream
Ingredients:
- Half a cup of cornstarch
- Half a cup of virgin coconut oil
- Eight drops of lavender essential oil
- Four drops of melaleuca oil
- Six drops of Roman chamomile essential oil

Instructions:
- Take a glass bowl and pour virgin coconut oil.
- Use an electric hand mixer to whip it until it makes stiff peaks.
- Now add lavender and Roman chamomile essential oil according to the mentioned ingredients.
- Add melaleuca oil only if your child is above the age of six months.
- Keep mixing until oils are distributed evenly.
- Add half a cup of cornstarch and stir it until a lotion-type consistency is obtained.
- Apply it to the affected area whenever you change your baby's diaper.

Recipe 2: Baking Soda Sponge Bath

Ingredients:
- 14 g of baking soda
- 235 ml of water

Instructions:
- Take a jar, pour water, and add baking soda into it.
- Close the jar and shake until the baking soda dissolves completely.
- Now, take a clean washcloth and soak it with the solution.
- Use this dampened cloth to cleanse the affected area of the baby's bottoms.
- Pat the area until it dries out.
- Use this solution to clean the rash area using a washcloth whenever you change the diaper.

DIARRHEA

According to UNICEF, Diarrhoea is a leading killer of children that kills around half a million children under five each year. Like constipation, Diarrhea is also a digestive problem. It is symptom of an infection in the gastrointestinal tract. In this condition, loose, watery, and continuous bowel movements occur. Diarrhea is also associated with other issues like vomiting, weight loss, nausea, and abdominal pain. **Danger signs that show you have diarrhea include fever, blood in the stool, mucus in the stool, vomiting, and bloating.** Generally, normal short-term diarrhea lasts for 1 or 2 days whereas prolonged long-term chronic diarrhea can last for several weeks.

NATURAL REMEDIES

1. **Plantain:** You can take plantain in the form of smoothies or juice. You can also take the leaves and seeds of this plant, chop them up, and steep them in cold water for a day.
2. **Goldenseal:** Goldenseal is a perfect remedy if your Diarrhea is caused by food poisoning or any digestive reaction. You can take it in the form of tea tincture.
3. **Myrrh and Geranium Essential Oil:** Take 1:1 of myrrh and geranium essential oils and blend them well. Take 16 drops of this solution over a day orally every half an hour. Don't take this for more than a day.
4. **Agrimony:** Make agrimony tea and take it four times per day.

Recipes for Treating Diarrhea

Recipe 1: Calming Capsule for Diarrhea
Ingredients:
- Six drops of black pepper essential oil
- Two drops of fennel essential oil
- Two drops of chamomile essential oil
- Two drops of peppermint essential oil
- One vegetable capsule
- Coconut oil

Instructions:
- Take a vegetable capsule and open it.
- Add all essential oils mentioned above, and top with coconut oil.
- Now, close the capsule gently.
- Take a capsule with coconut milk, water, or coconut water.

Recipe 2: Try Blackberry Tea
Ingredients:
- 710 ml of water
- 24 g of fresh honey
- 3 g of blackberry leaves (chopped and dried)

Instructions:
- First, take a saucepan and boil water in it.
- Add blueberry leaves to the saucepan.
- Remove the pan from the heat and cover it.
- Leave it steep for 20-25 minutes.
- Strain and discard the leaves.
- You can add honey to sweeten it according to your taste.

Recipe 3: Miso
Ingredients:
- 64 g of miso paste
- 475 ml of water
- Two minced garlic cloves
- 1 chopped scallion

Instructions:
- Take a bowl and add one spoon of miso paste to it.
- Boil water in a saucepan and reduce the heat to a low level.
- Take 60 ml of boiling water from the saucepan and pour into the bowl with miso.
- Stir it until miso and water combine well and attain a smooth texture.
- Now, add the mixture to the saucepan with the remaining water. Combine well.
- Add the one chopped scallion and stir continually.
- Turn off the heat.

- Add the minced garlic just before you take it.

DIZZINESS

It is a term that commonly refers to various sensations like **dizziness, weakness, inability to stand, and faintness**. In this condition, you will feel your surroundings spinning or moving.

NATURAL REMEDIES

1. **Orange Essential Oil:** Use this essential oil to ease your dizziness. You can use it in a diffuser or pour a few drops on your tissue and inhale.
2. **Indian Pink Flower Essence:** Take four drops of Indian pink flower essence under your tongue 2-4 times daily.
3. **Ginkgo and Hawthorn:** Take ginkgo and hawthorn 7-9 herbal capsules in combination daily or as needed.

Recipe for Treating Dizziness

Recipe: Stomach Settler Tea
Ingredients:
- 4 tsp of ginger
- Dashes of ground pumpkin seed
- Celery seed
- Chamomile Flowers
- Fennel
- Orange rind
- Peppermint
- Spearmint
- 2 cups of boiling water

Instructions:
- Take boiling water in a pan, and add ginger.
- Add all seeds and herbs.
- Cover the pan with a lid and steep for 15 - 20 minutes.
- Stain and drink the tea.

DRY EYES

Dry eyes are a common condition in which your tear glands produce unstable or poor-quality tears for your eyes. As a result, your eye's surface becomes inflamed and damaged. **The symptoms of dry eyes include eye redness, eye fatigue, stinging sensation, burning, difficulty with nighttime driving, and many more.**

NATURAL REMEDIES

1. **Chamomile:** Use chamomile to make an infusion. Use two cotton pads and soak them in solution. Leave these cotton pads on your eyes for rest and wait 10-15 minutes.

2. **Cornflower Water:** Take cornflower water and soak cotton pads in it. Leave these soaking pads on your eyes to rest and wait 10-15 minutes. Remove the pads and use clean water to rinse your eyes.

3. **Drink More Water:** Drinking more water helps you to keep your eyes moist. Don't just drink water; eat water-rich foods like watermelon, cucumbers, and coconut.

4. **Warm Compress:** Use a clean, lint-free cloth and soak it in warm water. Take it out and wring it, put this cloth on your eyes, and wait until it cools down. Repeat this process 4-5 times a day until you feel your eyes are getting better.

DRY MOUTH

In this condition, your mouth's salivary glands don't produce enough saliva to keep your mouth wet. Common causes of dry mouth can be side effects of certain medications or radiation therapy. Most people are affected by this condition in their old age. **You may notice these signs if your salivary glands are not producing enough saliva, such as dry mouth, bad breath, dry tongue, dry hoarseness, etc.**

NATURAL REMEDIES

1. **Aloe Vera:** Try aloe vera juice to treat your dry mouth. It is a great way to cure this condition because gel in aloe vera leaves moisturizes your mouth and stimulates saliva production.

2. **Marshmallow Root:** Like aloe vera, marshmallow root stimulates saliva production and relieves dry mouth.

3. **Frozen Melon:** Use a water-rich refreshing slice of melon between your gum and cheek for 1-2 hours. If this remedy helps and relieves dry mouth, use a small bag to keep some thinly sliced melons in the freezer. Repeat this remedy 2-3 times daily and use these frozen melons.

4. **Stay Hydrated:** Drinking more water helps you to keep your mouth hydrated. Besides drinking water, eat water-rich foods such as watermelon, cucumbers, and coconut.

DRY SKIN

In this condition, your skin feels scaly, rough, and itchy. People of all ages can be affected by this skin condition. The other medical terms used for this ailment are xerosis or xeroderma. Dry skin can result from using harsh soaps, overbathing, changes in weather, and sun damage.

NATURAL REMEDIES

1. **Chickweed-Aloe Gel:** Make chickweed-aloe gel to treat your dry skin. It nourishes your skin and gives it moisture. Apply this gel to your skin. It absorbs quickly and has no odor. You can make this gel and refrigerate it for up to two weeks.

2. **Coconut Oil:** Use coconut oil instead of soap to cleanse your face. Take a cotton swab and dab coconut oil on your eyes and all over your face to remove makeup. Now, use warm water to raise your face and pat it dry.

Recipe: Glistening Glycerol

Ingredients:
- 60 ml of boiled and cooled water
- Half tsp of vegetable glycerin
- Half tsp of avocado oil

Instructions:
- Take a small bowl, pour water and glycerin, and combine them well.
- Save this mixture in a sterile container and cover tightly.
- Before applying this moisturizer, wash your face gently.
- Apply this moisturizer all over your skin with clean fingertips.

EAR INFECTION

All three parts of the ear are sensitive to infection at certain ages or conditions. Bacteria, viruses, fungi, and yeast are infection-causing agents in the ear. **Signs of ear infection include hearing loss, dizziness, vomiting, and rapid involuntary eye movement.**

NATURAL REMEDIES

1. **Lavender Oil:** Pour 3-4 drops of lavender oil into your ear for pain relief. You can also mix this oil with thyme and almond for enhanced effects.
2. **Garlic Oil or Mullein Oil:** Mix these oils and add 2-4 drops to the infectious ear. That will provide long-term relief from the infection.
3. **Anti-Swimmer's Drops:** Mix equal rubbing alcohol and white vinegar and place 2-3 drops in both ears before and after swimming. Let the mixture reach the ear canal and then drain out. Their acidic pH will prevent microbial colonization while swimming.
4. **Olive Oil Drops:** Add 2-3 drops of slightly warm olive oil in the ear and leave for 10-15 minutes. It will help deal with the pain. Use it 3-4 times a day.

Recipe for Treating Ear Infection

Recipe: Herbal Ear Drops

Ingredients:
- 2 tbsp olive oil or coconut oil (carrier oil)
- 1 tsp mullein flower oil
- 1 tsp garlic-infused oil
- 1 tsp calendula oil
- 3-4 drops of tea tree essential oil
- 3-4 drops of lavender essential oil
- Glass dropper bottle

Instructions:

- Mix carrier, mullein flower, garlic-infused, and calendula oil. Let infuse for 24 hours.
- Strain the oils to remove plant matter.
- Add tea tree and lavender essential oils mix.
- Transfer to a dropper bottle.
- Add 2-3 drops to the affected ear.
- Lie down with the ear facing up for a few minutes.
- Gently massage around the ear to aid absorption.

ECZEMA

Atopic dermatitis affects the outer skin layer. **This condition results in skin inflammation, dryness, itching, bumpiness, thick red patches, and many more.** Eczema causing factors include allergens, dry or cold weather, or specific exposures. Eczema can come and go and can be seasonal for some individuals.

NATURAL REMEDIES

1. **Cardamom:** Blend cardamom to make powder. Use powder to make a paste in water or honey. Apply the paste/mask on the affected skin for 20-25 minutes for smooth skin.
2. **Calendula-Goldenseal Spray:** Take 1 ounce of dried goldenseal root, calendula each, ¾ cup witch hazel, and ¼ cup jojoba oil. Cook the dried herbs and jojoba oil on low flame for 3-5 hours. Strain the mixture and mix with witch hazel. Take a spray bottle, pour this in it, and spray on affected skin 2-3 times daily.
3. **Avocado Rub:** Take a peeled fresh avocado and make the finest paste. Rub this on the affected area and leave for 5 minutes. Wash or clean the area with a wet cloth.
4. **Coconut Rub:** Massage the oil on the affected area after a shower and leave. You can also use coconut butter as cream.
5. **Glistening Glycerol:** Mix half a tsp of vegetable glycerin in 60ml of boiled cool water. Add half a tsp of almond oil to the mixture. Apply this recipe to the affected area after washing.

Recipe for Treating Eczema

Recipe: Essence Oil for Dry Eczema

Ingredients:

- 6 tsp of rosehip seed oil
- 1 ml lavender oil
- 10ml Calophyllum oil
- 1ml palmarosa oil

Instructions:

- Take a clean glass bowl.
- Mix all the oils of the given quantity in a bowl.
- Pour this mixture into a clean glass bottle.

- Apply the mixture 3-4 times a day on dry eczema.
- This mixture will promote skin healing and ease itching.
- Combine the same quantity of seed oil and calophyllum oil with 1ml Eucalyptus citriodora and 1ml thyme oil for weeping eczema.

ELBOW PAIN

Elbow pain can be because of some injury or pain in joints, muscles, bones, alignment, or other issues. This pain can also affect the hand muscles with pain, numbness, weakening, swelling, aches, etc. **Other symptoms are:**

- Loss of grip.
- Swelling or bumping on the elbow area.
- Severe pain.
- Difficulty in arm and hand movement.

Long-term pain indicates severe issues and needs physician consultation.

NATURAL REMEDIES

1. **Turmeric:** Add one tsp in a glass of hot milk and drink once daily.
2. **Ginger:** You can consume ginger differently, like eating raw ginger, applying ginger paste, drinking ginger tea, etc. Avoid taking >4 grams of ginger per day.
3. **Hot and Cold Compress:** Both hot and cold compresses are effective for pain relief. Take a cloth and soak it in warm water. Squeeze extra water and compress the effective elbow with the material until it cools down. Avoid hot compress if the elbow is swollen. You can apply ice directly on the elbow for 10-20 minutes for a cold compress. It is best for both swelling and pain reduction.
4. **Essential Oils:** Mix a few drops of frankincense, peppermint, and carrier oil (almond oil) and apply on the affected elbow 3 times daily.

Recipe for Treating Elbow Pain

Recipe: Epsom Salt and Lavender Essential Oil Bath

Ingredients:

- 1/2 to 1 cup of Epsom salt
- 5-10 drops of lavender essential oil
- Warm bathwater

Instructions:

- Fill the bathtub with warm water. Maintain the water temperature to your comfort level.
- Add the Epsom salt to the water, and dissolve properly. This salt contains magnesium, a component that minimizes pain and relaxes muscles.
- Add 8-12 drops of lavender oil to the tub for soothing properties.
- Remain in the tub for 20-30 minutes for complete relaxation.
- Take this bath once a day until you feel better.

EYE SCRATCH

A scratch on the cornea, the white part inside the eye, is known as an eye scratch or corneal abrasion. As a scratch is superficial, it is not harmful but can be a serious issue if it develops infection. Any foreign particle that enters the eye or accident can cause a scratch. **The common signs of scratch are irritation, pain, tearing, blurriness, light sensitivity, and redness.**

NATURAL REMEDIES

1. **Coconut Oil:** Add a drop of coconut oil in a practical eye for 1-2 times daily. The oil helps with irritation and dryness and prevents infection. Coconut oil is entirely safe to use in the eyes.
2. **Chamomile Tea Compress:** Place the chamomile tea bag in hot water for 2-3 minutes. Let the tea bag cool down and press on the affected eye for 10-15 minutes. This compress will help the scratch heal faster. You can also use a green tea bag as a replacement.
3. **Cedarwood Oil:** Inhalation of cedarwood oil will help in pain reduction caused by eye scratches.
4. **Rose Water:** Add a few drops of rose water to the eye to prevent infection or reduce inflammation. You can also use the dipped cotton swab to keep the rose water in your eyes for a long time.
5. **Wear Glasses:** Scratching can make the eyes sensitive to light. So, the light can irritate, burn, or tear. Make sure to wear glass for light and dust protection.

<u>Recipe for Treating Eye Scratch</u>

Recipe: Honey Spray
Ingredients:
- 3 tbsp of honey
- 2 cups of water

Instruction:
- Add honey to boiling water.
- Let the mixture cool down.
- Splash the water on your eyes to relieve irritation, redness, or dryness.

EYESTRAIN

Eye strain is also known as asthenopia. The excessive use of eyes and ignoring of glasses, especially in precise work like computer use, reading, and stitching, cause fatigue of the eyes, also known as eyestrain. **This condition results in tearing, redness, burning, pain, sensitivity, loss of focus, itching of the eyes, and headache.** This condition can get better after a break to the eyes and rest. However, ignorance can lead you toward medications. The 20-20-20 rule is very helpful to prevent. The rule is very simple. While looking at something close-up then for every 20 minutes, look away to an object or anything approximately for a distance of 20 feet for at least 20 seconds.

NATURAL REMEDIES

1. **Chamomile Eyewash:** Make an infusion of 1 tsp of dried red raspberry leaves, 1 tsp of dried calendula, and 1sp of dried chamomile in water. After a few minutes, perfectly strain the infusion and wash your eyes with the strained water.

2. **Essential Oil:** Spray Green Myrtle hydrosol in your eyes six times each day to deal with eye redness, fatigue, and dryness. You can also use a byproduct, hydrosol, from distilling essential oils.

3. **Flower Essence:** Place the Wild Carrot flowers and Brodiaea elegans flowers in a bottle filled with spring water. Leave the water under the sun for 4-5 hours. Stain the water properly and fill in a spray bottle. Spray this flower essence into the affected eye to deal with dryness, fatigue, and redness.

4. **Cold Water Wash:** Cold water is best to increase blood circulation in any body area and helps relax tissues. Use cold water to wash your eyes to relieve fatigue and discomfort.

5. **Aloe Vera:** Apply cold aloe vera gel on your eyes for 10 minutes for relaxation, improved blood circulation, and puffiness.

<u>Recipe for Treating Eye Strain</u>

Recipe: Eyestrain-Relief Berry Smoothie

Ingredients:

- 1 cup mixed berries (blueberries, strawberries, raspberries)
- One ripe banana
- Half a cup of spinach leaves (fresh or frozen)
- Half cup plain Greek yogurt
- Half a cup of any milk of your choice
- One tbsp honey (optional for sweetness)
- 1 tsp chia seeds (optional, for added nutrients)

Instructions:

- Wash and peel the fruits.
- Add all the ingredients in a blender and make a smooth mixture.
- Maintain the consistency with almond milk.
- Add honey to maintain sweetness.
- Take this smoothie once a day to relieve eye strain and improve eyesight.

FATIGUE

Fatigue is associated with mental and physical tiredness, exhaustion, and lack of energy. **Its signs are dizziness, weakness of muscles, muscle aches and soreness, delayed responses, and anxiety.** Reasons for fatigue are excessive workload, depression, lack of dietary nutrients, being overweight, etc. A few lifestyle changes can minimize fatigue, but if it is long-term, you must consult the physician because it can be associated with some severe disease.

NATURAL REMEDIES

1. **Essential Oils:** Add a drop of Thyme oil, Peppermint oil, two drops of orange oil, and three drops of Rosemary in a tub of warm water. Relax your body in the bathtub for 20-30 minutes, and you will feel fresh.
2. **Electrolyte Drinks:** These drinks are rich in minerals and can also compensate for the water deficiency in your body. Both water and mineral deficiency can also cause fatigue, so you can try these drinks to gain energy.
3. **Fresh Purified Water:** Add a few cucumber slices, mint leaves, and lemon slices to your water bottle. Mint and cucumber contain antimicrobial properties; lemon is antioxidant and rich in Vitamin C, which will help the body against infections.
4. **Spanish:** Spanish contains many valuable compounds like Vitamin B and potassium, which produce energy in the body. Make sure to add a handful of Spanish to your daily diet.
5. **Drumstick Leaves or Aloe Vera Gel:** Consume half a tsp of aloe vera gel with a bit of turmeric or add 2 tsp of drumstick leaves in a cup of milk. Boil and strain the milk and drink once a day.

Recipe for Treating Fatigue

Recipe: Licorice-Rosemary Syrup

Ingredients:

- 2 tbsp dried licorice root
- 1 tbsp dried rosemary leaves
- 3 cups water
- 1 cup honey (adjust to taste)
- Cheesecloth or fine mesh strainer
- Glass jar or bottle for storage

Instructions:

- Add dried rosemary leaves and licorice root in a pot with water.
- Place the pot on a medium flame for 20-30 minutes till the water remains half.
- Strain the water with cheesecloth.
- Add the desired amount of honey for sweetness.
- Store the syrup in a sterilized bottle.
- Take 1-2 tsp of syrup directly or add in warm water.
- Consume once a day.
- Avoid giving kids.

FEVER

Fever is the body's natural defence against infection or illness. It is an increase in body temperature that helps clear foreign agents inside the body. **Sweating, dehydration, general weakness, and loss of appetite are common symptoms of fever.**

NATURAL REMEDIES

1. **Pineapple:** Take a few bites of fresh pineapple after every 1-2 hours. Do not use canned pineapple.
2. **Linden Tea:** Mix the powder of dry chamomile flowers, linden flowers, and thyme. Add one tsp of powder to a hot boiled water cup. Leave for 5 minutes and strain the water. Drink this tea a few times a day.
3. **Essential Oils:** When diluted in a carrier oil, some essential oils, like eucalyptus and lavender, can be applied to the skin for cooling sensations and comfort. Inhalation of these oils may also provide relief from fever.
4. **Cool Compress:** Soak the washcloth in cool water, wring it out, and place it on your forehead, wrists, or neck. You can also wear the frozen soaks that will work the same.

Recipe for Treating Fever

Recipe: Blushing Apple Smoothie

Ingredients:
- Two medium apples, peeled, cored, and chopped
- 1 cup fresh strawberries, hulled
- 1/2 cup plain yogurt
- 1/2 cup coconut water or water
- One tablespoon honey (adjust to taste)
- Ice cubes (optional)

Instructions:
- Wash the fruits and peel the apples.
- Add apples and strawberries in a blender with coconut water and yogurt.
- Blend until a smooth, creamy mixture forms.
- Add honey if you want sweetness.
- Have a glass of smoothie every day.
- It will boost your immune system, hydrate the body, and replenish electrolytes to treat fever.

FLU

Flu is known as a contagious infection caused by influenza viruses. There are two main types of these viruses: type A and type B. **Type A is more prevalent with symptoms like coughing, sneezing, sore throat, chills, and fever. Type B virus is more common in kids and shows chills, respiratory symptoms, and high fever.** As viruses cause the flu, antibiotics cannot be its cure, but some home remedies can help you.

NATURAL REMEDIES

1. **Essential Oils:** Mix one part of lavender, rosewood, lemon, and eucalyptus oil, each with three pieces of Ravensara oil. Use this mixture as a diffuser, massage, or to take a bath if you have the flu.

2. **Ginger:** You can drink ginger tea twice daily for the flu. Take 2-3 grams of ginger and only 1 gram daily if pregnant.

3. **Garlic:** Eat 3-4 cloves of raw garlic twice daily to reduce flu symptoms and quick recovery.

4. **Licorice Roots Syrup:** Licorice has impressive properties against the flu, like easing pain, nasal passage clearance, relaxing chest congestion, suppressing cough, and relieving sore throat. Add Licorice roots to a glass and fill the glass with water. Leave the soaked seeds for 3-4 hours and strain the water. Add honey in water for sweetness. Store the syrup in a sterile bottle and 1 tsp every few hours.

5. **Catnip-Hyssop Tea:** If you are feeling body aches or sore throat because of the flu, one cup of Catnip-Hyssop tea will relax your body and boost the immune system. Add one tsp of dry hyssop and one tsp of dry catnip in 1.5 cups of boiling water. Boil for 10 minutes till the water remains in one cup. Strain the tea and drink.

Important Note: This tea is not recommended for pregnant women.

Recipe for Treating Flue

Recipe: Goldenseal + Echinacea + Garlic Syrup

Ingredients:

- 1 tablespoon of dried goldenseal root
- 6-8 garlic cloves, crushed or minced
- One tablespoon of dried echinacea root
- 3 cups water
- 1 cup honey
- Cheesecloth or fine mesh strainer
- Glass jar or bottle for storage

Instructions:

- Add goldenseal, Echinacea, and garlic in a pan with water and leave on low flame for 30-40 minutes.
- Let the mixture cool down and strain with cheesecloth in a bowl.
- Add the strained liquid to the pan again and start adding honey.
- Stir until the honey is mixed in the mixture thoroughly.
- Transfer the mixture to a sterile jar or bottle and store it in the refrigerator.
- Take 1-2 tsp of syrup per day for flu symptoms.
- Pregnant women should avoid taking the syrup.

FOOD POISONING

Food poisoning is type of foodborne illness that children and adults get from something they ate or drank. A condition caused by eating undercooked or contaminated food is known as food poisoning. **Food poisoning symptoms are usually vomiting, fever, nausea, Diarrhea, and abdominal cramps.**

1. **Green Tea:** Add one tsp of lemon juice and honey to a cup of green tea. Both honey and lemon will boost your immune system.
2. **Rehydration Drink:** Continuous vomiting can cause food poisoning. It would help if you took as much liquid as you can. To rehydrate your body, mix two cups of water with ¼ cup of fresh orange juice, 2 tsp of honey, and ¼ tsp of baking soda. Have this drink once or twice a day.
3. **Barley Water:** To make this water:
   - ☐ Cook ¼ cup of raw barley in 710 ml of water on low flame for 1 hour.
   - ☐ Strain the water and let it cool down.
   - ☐ Add one tsp of honey or one pinch of salt, according to your preference.
4. **Apple Cider Vinegar:** Add one tsp of vinegar to a glass of water and drink it. It will help adjust the pH of your stomach.
5. **Ginger:** Make yourself a cup of ginger tea by steeping fresh ginger slices in hot water or sucking on ginger candies.
6. **Apple Gel:** Cook two unpeeled apples in half a cup of water. Also, add ¼ tsp of ground cinnamon and 1 tsp of honey. Cinnamon and honey will show the antibacterial effects. After 10 minutes, the apples will become soft. Eat these apples 1-2 times a day.

Recipe for Treating Food Poisoning

Recipe: Chicken Soup
Ingredients:
- One whole chicken (about 3-4 pounds)
- 10 cups of water
- Two carrots, peeled and chopped
- Two celery stalks, chopped
- One onion, chopped
- Three cloves garlic, minced
- One bay leaf
- Salt and pepper to taste
- Fresh parsley, chopped (for garnish)
- Cooked white rice (optional)

Instruction:
- Rinse chicken and place in a large pot with 10 cups of water.
- Bring to a boil, then simmer.
- Add chopped vegetables and season them with salt and pepper.
- Simmer for 1.5-2 hours until the chicken is tender.
- Remove the chicken, shred it, and strain the soup.
- Return broth, add chicken, and heat.
- Serve with optional rice and garnish with parsley.

FOOT AND ANKLE PAIN

There can be several reasons for pain in this area, like fatigue, injury, sprain, muscle stretch, etc. To relieve pain, you must try some natural remedies before taking medications. **Pain, swelling, and redness are common symptoms of this ailment.**

NATURAL REMEDIES

1. **Apple Cider Vinegar:** Add one cup of vinegar in 6 cups of warm water and soak your feet for half an hour to relieve pain.
2. **Essential Oil:** Use any of the essential oils to massage your feet and ankles daily. Massage will increase the blood circulation and reduce the pain after a few days.
3. **Cold and Warm Compress:** The cold and warm compress help relieve pain but are used in different conditions. Cold compress is usually used to minimize inflammation by reducing the blood flow. This compress is best for areas around tendons and joints. Take a frozen element like cloth, vegetable, or frozen bottle and compress the affected area for 15-20 minutes. You can repeat this process twice a day. A warm compress is similar to a cold compress. However, adding a cup of Epsom salt in warm water and placing your feet in water for 15-20 minutes will enhance the effect. A warm compress increases the blood flow and improves the healing process.
4. **RICE Therapy:** RICE therapy consists of 4 steps:
   - Rest
   - Ice
   - Compression
   - Elevation.

This therapy will protect your feet and ankle from swelling and speed healing.

Recipe for Treating Foot and Ankle Pain

Recipe: Cucumber Mint Foot Mask
Ingredients:
- Fresh Cucumber
- Fresh Mint Leaves
- Plain Yogurt
- Oatmeal
- Honey

Instructions:
- Blend half of the cucumber and a handful of mint leaves to paste.
- Mix 2 tbsp cucumber-mint paste, 2 tbsp plain yogurt, and 2 tbsp oatmeal in a bowl.
- Apply the mixture evenly on your feet and massage gently.
- Wrap your feet with plastic wrap and relax for 15-20 minutes.
- Remove the wrap, wipe off the mask, and soak feet in warm water for 5-10 mins.
- Pat feet dry and moisturize with lotion.
- Elevate your feet and unwind.

FOOT ODOR

Foot Odor is quite a common problem, because our feet sweat more than most other parts of the body because there are more sweat glands in the feet comparing to other body parts. Smelly feet (bromodosis) is when excessive sweating produces an unpleasant smell in socks and shoes. Other than the smell, sweating favors fungus growth and many other infection-causing microbes. The infection or fungal growth worsens the feet' smell. **Severe sweating is the most common symptom of foot odor.**

NATURAL REMEDIES

1. **Baking Powder:** Mix ¼ cup of cornstarch and ¼ cup of baking soda in a tray. Apply the mixture to your shoes and feet. The cornstarch will absorb the sweating, while baking soda eliminates the smell.
2. **Apple Cider Vinegar - Lavender Wash:** Add six drops of lavender oil in 60 ml vinegar and put the mixture in a spray bottle. Spray this mixture a few minutes before wearing the shoes.
3. **Coconut Tea Tree Deodorizer:** Mix 14g melted beeswax into 28g coconut oil. Add 2 tsp of cornstarch, 2 tsp of baking soda, and 3-4 drops of essential oil in the mixture. Store the mixture in a sterile bottle. The mixture will solidify after cooling down. Apply it as a moisturizer on your feet.
4. **Hydro Solution:** Mix 5 ml of hydrogen peroxide in a cup of water. Apply this solution to the odor areas once a day.

<u>Recipe for Treating Foot Odor</u>

Recipe: Essential Oil Foot Odor Spray

Ingredients:
- 1/2 cup distilled water
- 1 tbsp witch hazel
- Ten drops of tea tree oil
- Five drops of peppermint oil
- Five drops of lavender oil
- Five drops of eucalyptus oil

Instructions:
- First, mix witch hazel and water in a small bowl.
- Add all essential oils to the water mixture and stir well.
- Add the solution to the spray bottle by using a funnel.
- Apply the solution on your feet multiple times a day.

GAS, BELCHING, AND BLOATING

The collection of gas in the gastrointestinal tract results in gas, belching, and bloating. Typically, gas produced during digestion and belching expel gas from the stomach through the mouth. Bloating is a feeling of fullness in the abdomen due to excess gas or other factors. **The common signs are abdominal discomfort/pain, abdominal cramps, burping, flatulence, and others.** These symptoms can result from dietary choices, eating habits, or underlying medical conditions like IBS or constipation.

NATURAL REMEDIES

1. **Cinnamon:** Drink cinnamon or have a glass of milk with a tsp of cinnamon and honey.
2. **Peppermint:** Take 1-2 oil capsules before lunchtime or drink peppermint tea twice daily. It will relax the muscles of your gastrointestinal tract.
3. **Chamomile Tea:** Add one tsp of dried chamomile in boiling water. Steep for a few minutes, and strain the tea. Add honey if required, and drink twice a day.
4. **Fennel Seeds:** Chewing fennel seeds is an effective and quick way to deal with stomach cramps and gas. The volatile oil in these seeds promotes bile production, which helps in better digestion. You can add these seeds to your tea, too.
5. **Essential Oils:** You can use the essential oil massage to relieve the bloating, gas pain, and stomach cramps. Mix one tsp of vegetable oil with three drops of peppermint and two drops of cardamom oil and massage the abdominal area.

Recipe for Treating Gas, Belching, and Bloating

Recipe: Cucumber and Tomato Digestive Salad
Ingredients:
- Two medium cucumbers, thinly sliced
- Two medium tomatoes, diced
- 1/4 red onion, thinly sliced
- 1/4 cup fresh parsley, chopped
- One tablespoon extra-virgin olive oil
- One tablespoon of lemon juice
- One teaspoon of apple cider vinegar (optional)
- Salt and pepper to taste

Instructions:
- Slice cucumbers, dice tomatoes, and chop parsley.
- Mix cucumbers, tomatoes, onion, and parsley.
- Whisk olive oil and lemon juice together.
- Drizzle dressing over veggies and toss gently.
- Add salt and pepper to taste.
- Refrigerate for 15-30 mins.
- Serve as a light and refreshing salad.

GOUT

The type of arthritis caused by excessive uric acid production in the body is called gout. Due to metabolic disorders, purine is converted into uric acid stored in tissues and joints. **Gout symptoms are redness, swelling, severe pain in joints, restricted movement, and discomfort.** The major causes of gout are overeating, being overweight, alcohol consumption, a purine-rich diet, etc.

NATURAL REMEDIES

1. **Cherries:** According to NCBI research, eating 10-40 cherries reduces the painful attacks of gout by up to 35%. At the same time, combining allopurinol with cherries minimizes the risk by up to 75%.
2. **Vitamin C Intake:** Vitamin C can help bring down the uric acid level in the blood. As uric acid is the main reason for gout attacks, vitamin C can control this flash up to 44%. So, make sure to eat vitamin C-rich fruits and vegetables.
3. **Nettle Tea:** Nettle tea is rich in nutrients and serves as a cleaning agent to remove excessive waste from the body, such as uric acid. Take 1-3 cups of tea to deal with the swelling and pain of gout.
4. **Lavender Oil:** Dilute 4-5 drops of lavender oil with a carrier oil and slowly massage the affected area. You can also do it with vegetable oil.
5. **Rosemary Oil:** Rosemary oil may help improve circulation and reduce inflammation. Dilute and massage onto the affected joint.

<u>Recipe for Treating Gout</u>

Recipe: Ginger-Turmeric Gout Relief Tea
Ingredients:
- 1-inch piece of fresh ginger, sliced
- One teaspoon of ground turmeric
- One teaspoon of raw honey (optional)
- Juice of half a lemon
- 2 cups water

Instructions:
- Bring two cups of water to a boil in a pot.
- Once the water starts boiling, add the sliced ginger and ground turmeric. These ingredients have anti-inflammatory properties and help to flush the uric acid from the blood, which can help alleviate gout symptoms.
- Reduce the heat to a low level, cover the pot, and let it simmer for about 8-10 minutes.
- After simmering, strain the tea into a cup or mug. Discard the ginger and turmeric solids.
- Stir in raw honey for sweetness and a squeeze of lemon juice. Honey can add a touch of sweetness, while lemon juice provides vitamin C and antioxidants.

HAIR LOSS

Many people do not understand that it is very normal to lose 50 to 100 hairs every day, as new hair grows and replaces old hair. Hair loss happens due to an imbalance of hair growth and hair shedding. However, less and no new hair growth causes the thinning of hair or hair loss. **Its symptoms include bald patches on the scalp, complete body hair loss, and sudden hair loss.** It can be caused by genetics, aging, disease, hormonal imbalances, mineral deficiencies, and using improper hair products.

NATURAL REMEDIES

1. **Nasturtium Hair Rinse:** To make nasturtium hair rinse, add a cup of nasturtium leaves, ¼ cup of nettle, and rosemary leaves, each in 2 cups of apple vinegar, in a jar. Tightly close the pot and let the leaves steep for about a month. After a month, blend all the ingredients, and your hair rinse is ready. Apply this tincture to your hair after washing.

2. **Lavender-Rosemary Conditioner:** This conditioner will provide healthy and thick hair by keeping your scalp well-nourished. Mix 1.5 ml of rosemary oil, 0.75 ml of lavender oil, a cup of melted sunflower oil, and one cup of melted cocoa butter to make the conditioner. Apply the one tbsp of conditioner after shampooing, leave for half a minute, and then rinse. Apply it for a month, and you'll notice a clear difference.

3. **Eclipta Alba:** According to recent research, Eclipta is effective for hair growth even more than minoxidil. Massage the Eclipta extract on your scalp. Avoid taking the section orally.

4. **Garlic:** To apply garlic to the scalp, crush 5-6 cloves, mix with an essential oil like coconut, and massage on the scalp for half an hour.

5. **Nettle Extract:** To make the extract, boil nettle leaves in water for 10 minutes. Strain the water, cool down, and use it to rinse the hair.

Recipe for Treating Hair Loss

Recipe: Ginkgo-Rosemary Tonic

Ingredients:
- 2 tbsp coconut oil
- 1 cup witch hazel
- 14g dried ginkgo biloba leaves
- 14g dried rosemary leaves

Instructions:
- Add coconut oil and herbs to a cooker. Let the herbs steep for 3-5 hours on low flame.
- Let the oil cool down and strain properly with cheesecloth.
- Add the oil to the bottle and mix with one cup of witch hazel.
- Spray the tonic on the hair loss area 1-2 times after hair wash and massage. Apply it 1-2 times daily.

HANGOVER

A combination of symptoms that results in excessive alcohol intake is known as hangover. **The common symptoms include vomiting, thirst, weakness, headache, dizziness, heartburn, fatigue, and dry mouth.** The increased and drastically decreased blood sugar levels due to excessive drinking cause these symptoms. It takes about 24 hours maximum to deal with these symptoms altogether. However, some natural remedies can help you deal with the symptoms quickly.

NATURAL REMEDIES

1. **Barberry Berries Tea:** Add one tsp of Oregon grape root and one tsp of ripe barberry in two cups of boiling water. Let the ingredients soak for half an hour, then strain the water. Drink a cup of this water once a day.
2. **Peppermint, Chaparral, Catnip Tea:** Boil one tsp leaves of each in 2 cups of water and steep for 20-30 minutes. Stain the water and enjoy a cup of your tea.
3. **Prickly Pear:** According to clinical trials, consuming prickly pear before alcohol consumption reduces the risk of hangover symptoms by up to 50%. Consume one tbsp of prickly pear hangover terminator five hours before drinking.
4. **Bananas:** Bananas are rich in magnesium and potassium, which help deal with hangover symptoms like fatigue and nausea within a half hour. Alcohol removes these minerals from the body so that bananas will replenish your body.
5. **Honey:** Take a few tsp of raw honey or mix it with the tea or water and take it early in the morning.
6. **Tomato:** Like honey, tomatoes also help your system clean from remaining alcohol and provide essential nutrients to the body that are lost due to drinking. Drink tomato juice early in the morning.

Recipe for Treating Hangover

Recipe: Natural Hangover Relief Elixir
Ingredients:
- 1 cup coconut water
- 1 tsp honey
- 1 tsp fresh lemon juice
- 1/4 tsp ginger (grated or powdered)
- A pinch of turmeric
- A pinch of salt
- Optional: a few mint leaves

Instructions:
- Take a class and mix all the ingredients: lemon juice, coconut water, honey, ginger, and salt.
- Cut the mint leaves and add to the mixture. Mint will help you with nausea.
- Drink this elixir in the morning to keep your body hydrated.

HEADACHE

Unfortunately, there are roughly around 45 million Americans feel headaches each year. It is estimated that each day, 15.8% of the world's population had headache. The common causes of headaches are tension, stress, sinus issues, dehydration, eyestrain, and migraines. **The common symptoms are irritability, nausea, pain in the back and shoulders, ringing in the ear, and slow headache onset.**

NATURAL REMEDIES

1. **Tincture Blend:** Mix 2 tbsp of willow, 1 tbsp of basil, and peppermint tincture in a dropper bottle. Add 1-2 dropperfuls of water and juice. Take this blend every half hour 2-3 times until you feel better.

2. **Peppermint Compress:** You can apply peppermint oil to your forehead for headaches or make your herbal compress. Compress steep peppermint tea bags into two cups of boiling water for half an hour to make this. Remove the herb bags and add the ice cube to the water. Take a soft cloth, soak it in water, and press on your forehead. Repeat until you feel better.

3. **Herbal Tea:** To make the infusion, mix half a cup of dried marshmallow leaves and linden leaves each, one cup of dried meadowsweet flower and betony leaf each, and ¼ cup of lettuce stalk and leaves. Steep 2-3 tbsp of herbal mix in boiling water for half an hour and drink the water.

4. **Eucalyptus:** If you feel any signs of headache, mix eucalyptus and peppermint oil on your palm. Apply this mixture on the sides of your head and behind the ear. You can apply again after an hour.

5. **Butterbur:** According to studies, butterbur extract is effective against migraine attacks. A person should take 75 mg orally twice daily to relieve migraine.

6. **Coffee:** Mix ¼ tsp of cinnamon, 2 tbsp honey, ¼ tsp of vanilla extract, and 60ml non-dairy milk in your freshly brewed coffee for headache treatment.

7. **Ice Compress:** Compress frozen gel or ice pack on the pain area for 10 minutes for pain relief.

Recipe for Treating Headache

Recipe: Bay Leaf Broth

Ingredients:
- 4-5 dried bay leaves
- One small onion, chopped
- Two cloves of garlic, minced
- 4 cups of water
- One tablespoon of olive oil
- Salt and pepper to taste

Instructions:

- Heat the olive oil in a saucepan and sauté onion and garlic until golden brown.
- Add dry bay leaf and Sauté for another minute.
- Add water and boil.
- Add salt and pepper and steep the broth on low flame for half an hour.
- Strain the broth and mesh the strained onion, garlic, and leaves. Remix them with the broth and serve.

HEARTBURN

Many people experience discomfort in their digestive system followed by a burning sensation or discomfort in their chest or throat. It is often caused by stomach acid moving up into the esophagus. This acid causes damage and inflammation in the esophagus walls. Various factors trigger heartburn, like GERD, spicy food, excessive alcohol or coffee intake, stress, lying down after eating, etc. **Common symptoms of heartburn are difficulty swallowing, sour/acidic taste in mouth, burning sensation, and vomiting.**

NATURAL REMEDIES

1. **Ginger Tea:** To prepare the tea:
   - Boil 1 tsp of chopped ginger in two cups of water for 10 minutes until the water remains half.
   - Add honey to sweeten your drink of tea.
   - Avoid ginger tea if you have bleeding problems, gallbladder, or high blood pressure issues.
2. **Fennel-Angelica Syrup:** Steep 1 tbsp of fennel seeds and one ounce of dry angelica in two cups of water. Strain the mixture with cheesecloth when the water remains half. Pour the liquid into the pan again and add two cups of honey. Stir well, and your syrup is ready. Store the syrup in a glass bottle. You can take one tbsp of this syrup three times/day.
3. **Potatoes:** Chewing raw potato slices or diluted potato juice shows tremendous effects against heartburn in less than 30 minutes.
4. **Basil:** Chew 2-3 fresh basil leaves early in the morning to treat heartburn. Remember, dry leaves are not effective.
5. **Almonds:** Eat a handful of almonds to improve digestion and reduce heartburn.
6. **Chamomile:** Add one tbsp of dried chamomile to a cup of water and steep for 15-20. The addition of garlic or lemon will enhance the effects.
7. **Marshmallow Roots:** You can use 2-4 tbsp of dried roots to make tea.

Recipe for Treating Heartburn

Recipe: Banana Oatmeal Smoothie
Ingredients:

- One ripe banana
- 1/2 cup old-fashioned oats

- 1 cup unsweetened almond milk
- 1/2 tsp ground cinnamon
- 1 tsp chia seeds (optional)
- 1 tsp honey (optional)

Instructions:

- Blend banana, oats, almond milk, cinnamon, and chia seeds (if using) until smooth.
- Add honey for sweetness if required.
- Have a glass of this smoothie once a day.
- Banana suppresses acid production in the stomach, while oat absorbs the acidic stomach. Together, both of these relieve the heartburn.

HEAT EXHAUSTION

High temperature, continuous hard work, and insufficient liquid intake can cause heat exhaustion. **The common symptoms are fatigue, dizziness, nausea, sweating, and increased heart rate.** If not treated on time, heat exhaustion can lead to life-threatening heatstroke. So, it's essential to keep your body hydrated.

NATURAL REMEDIES

1. **Hydration:** In case you feel any symptoms of heat exhaustion, drink water immediately. The electrolyte-rich drinks are even better for such conditions to replenish the body's water and minerals together. A person should drink 10-15 cups of water on average.
2. **Peppermint and Chamomile:** Consume 2-3 cups of iced peppermint and chamomile tea a day for heat exhaustion.
3. **Sage Iced Tea:** You can consume 3-6 cups of sage iced tea to save yourself from heat exhaustion and hot flashes. To make the tea, steep 1 tbsp of sage leaves in water for 5-10 minutes.
4. **Lemon:** Squeeze fresh lemon juice into a cup of water, add salt and a teaspoon of honey, and drink this mixture to stay hydrated and balanced.
5. **Sandalwood:** Mix sandalwood powder with some water to make a paste and apply it to your forehead and neck. Leave it on until it dries, then wash off with cool water.

Recipe for Treating Heat Exhaustion

Recipe: Watermelon and Cucumber Hydration Salad

Ingredients:

- 2 cups cubed watermelon (chilled)
- One cucumber (peeled and sliced)
- 1 tbsp fresh lime juice
- 1 tbsp fresh mint leaves (chopped)
- A pinch of black salt or sea salt (for electrolytes)
- Freshly ground black pepper (to taste)

Instructions:

- Cut the watermelon and cucumber into cubes. Let the watermelon cool down in the refrigerator for about an hour.
- Add cucumber and watermelon in a large bowl and mix with 1 tbsp of lime juice.
- Add chopped mint leaves, a pinch of salt, and black pepper.
- Mix all the ingredients and serve.

HEEL PAIN

Heel discomfort can occur for various reasons, including plantar fasciitis, obesity, walking or leaping on rough or hard surfaces, wearing uncomfortable or improperly fitted shoes, illness, or accident. **Symptoms include sensitivity, inflammation, stiffness, discoloration, and bumps on heels.**

NATURAL REMEDIES

1. **Epsom Salt Soak:** Add a cup of Epsom salt to a basin of warm water and soak your feet for 15-20 minutes. Epsom salt can help reduce inflammation and relax the muscles.
2. **Cold Compress:** Grab a frozen water bottle and place it under your feet. Spend around five minutes gently rolling your feet on the bottle.
3. **Turmeric Paste:** Use a little coconut oil and turmeric powder to make a paste. Apply this paste to the troublesome heel, dry it, and thoroughly rinse.
4. **Ginger Compress:** Ginger should be grated fresh, wrapped in a cloth, and soaked in boiling water. For 15 to 20 minutes, apply the warm ginger compress to the sore area.
5. **Essential Oils:** Any essential oil including those from eucalyptus, peppermint, rosemary, and lavender, is acceptable. Massage your heels with one tablespoon of carrier oil and two or three drops of essential oil.
6. **Apple Cider Vinegar Soak:** Add one cup of vinegar to six glasses of warm water. Soak your feet in water for 10 to 20 minutes.

Recipe for Treating Heel Pain

Recipe: Heel Pain Relief Salve
Ingredients:

- 1/4 cup coconut oil
- 2 tbsp beeswax pellets
- Ten drops of peppermint oil
- Ten drops of lavender oil
- Ten drops of eucalyptus oil
- Five drops of tea tree oil

Instructions:

- Put a glass bowl made of heat-resistant material in a pan of boiling water.
- Beeswax and coconut oil should be added to the bowl and let it melt.
- Let the beeswax and coconut oil cool slightly when they have adequately melted.

- Mix well after adding the essential oils to the mixture.
- After cooling, pour the contents into a glass bottle that has been sterilized.
- Massage your heels with a tiny bit of the balm.

HICCUPS

Hiccups/ hiccoughs/ singultus are uncontrollable and repeated contraction of the diaphragm or glottis muscles that produce a "hic" sound. **Other symptoms include stomach and chest tightening and stomach spasms.** Hiccups can be caused by swallowing air, excessive eating or drinking, stress or anxiety, irritated nerves, low blood CO_2 levels, and being emotional or excited.

NATURAL REMEDIES

1. **Essential Oils:**
   - Sniffing **sandalwood oil** will calm your hiccups in case of anxiety or stress.
   - **Peppermint oil** calms lower esophageal sphincter, which helps stop hiccups.
   - **Basil oil** helps relax muscle spasms, which is the actual cause of hiccups.
   - **Tarragon oil** can immediately stop hiccoughs by relaxing neuromuscular spasms.

   You can use any of these oils available. Sniff the oil directly from the bottle or sprinkle it on a tissue to sniff it.
2. **Honey or Sugar:** Honey stops the hiccups by calming the vagus nerve that interrupts hiccups to relax. In contrast, the sugar granules disturb spasms in the diaphragm by causing throat irritation.
3. **Breathing in Paper Bag:** Breathing in a paper bag can calm the hiccups caused by low levels of CO_2 in the blood.

Recipe for Treating Hiccups

Recipe: Calming Hiccup Tea

Ingredients:
- 1 tsp chamomile flowers (dried)
- 1/2 tsp fennel seeds
- 1/2 tsp lemon balm leaves (dried)
- 1 cup hot water
- Honey to taste

Instructions:
- Add chamomile flowers, fennel seeds, and lemon balm leaves in a bowl.
- Pour a cup of boiling water over the herbal mix. Cover the cup for five to ten minutes and allow the herbs to steep.
- After steeping, filter the tea to remove the herbal solids and pour it into a fresh cup.
- Add a bit of honey to sweeten the tea, if preferred.
- Sip the tea carefully while allowing it to cool slightly. The diaphragm may be relaxed by the warm environment and calming herbs.

HIGH BLOOD PRESSURE

It is a medical condition characterized by high blood pressure in blood arteries. This high pressure damages the blood vessels and decreases the oxygen and blood flow toward the heart, which can cause heart damage. The common causes of hypertension include obesity, diabetes, stress, high cholesterol levels, smoking, and more. **Its symptoms are headache, nausea, dizziness, blurry vision, chest pain, and ringing in the ears.**

NEW GUIDELINE FROM THE AMERICAN HEART ASSOCIATION:

Blood Pressure Categories	SYSTOLIC mm HG (Upper Number)		DIASTOLIC mm HG (Lower Number)
Normal	Less than 120	and	Less than 80
Elevated	120-129	and	Less than 80
High Blood Pressure (HYPERTENTION) STAGE 1	130-139	or	80-89
High Blood Pressure (HYPERTENTION) STAGE 2	140 or Higher	or	90 OR HIGHER
Hypertensive Crisis (Consult your Doctor Immediately)	Higher than 180	and /or	HIGHER THAN 120

NATURAL REMEDIES

1. **Green Tea:** You can take 1-3 cups of tea daily to keep yourself fresh the whole day.
2. **Lavender Oil:** You can inhale the oil directly from the bottle or mix it with carrier oil to add room freshener. However, taking lavender oil in combination with medication can lower your BP too much, so be careful.
3. **Turmeric:** You can consume turmeric in tea, juice, or adding in milk.
4. **Pomegranate:** According to a study in 2012, taking a cup of pomegranate juice for about a month might reduce hypertension in the short term. This fruit is rich in nutrients and antioxidants that might stop high blood pressure.
5. **Flaxseeds:** Add ground flax seeds to smoothies, yogurt, or oatmeal. Start with 1-2 tablespoons daily and gradually increase the amount if desired.
6. **Alfalfa:** Many compounds in alfalfa lower blood pressure by relaxing blood vessels. You can add alfalfa to your routine sandwiches or salads.
7. **Garlic:** Consume fresh/cooked garlic into your meals. A typical recommended dose is one to two cloves per day.

Recipe for Treating High Blood Pressure

Recipe: Cocoa Smoothie

Ingredients:

- 2-3 tbsp natural cocoa powder
- 1 tsp flax seeds

- 1 tbsp honey
- 1 cup almond milk
- One banana

Instructions:

- Blend all the ingredients until you'll get a smooth texture.
- Adjust the smoothness by increasing or decreasing the almond milk amount.
- The addition of honey is optional.
- You can take 1-2 servings of this smoothie.

HIGH CHOLESTEROL

Cholesterol is a part of many body tissues, but its high concentration in blood can be problematic. High cholesterol can be caused by being overweight, less physical work, disease, smoking/drinking, and eating high-fat food. **This condition has no visible symptoms, but its effect on other organs can lead to severe stroke or heart attack.**

NATURAL REMEDIES

1. **Vitamin B5:** Vitamin B5/pantothenic acid shows effective results in lowering blood cholesterol levels. You can eat foods rich in vitamin B5, avocado, cereals, seeds, nuts, etc.
2. **Garlic:** Based on studies, eating 3-6 grams of garlic lowers blood cholesterol by 10% for eight weeks.
3. **Stanols and Plant Sterols:** These elements are present in some fortified meals. **How Much:** Include 2-3 grams of plant sterols or stanols in your diet each day.
4. **Leaf Tea :** Consume two to three cups of green tea each day for potential advantages.
5. **Veggies and Fruits:** Consume five servings or more of fruits and vegetables daily to decrease cholesterol.
6. **Legumes:** Soluble fiber and plant-based protein are abundant in legumes, which can help decrease LDL cholesterol. Include beans or lentils multiple times in your meals a week.

<u>Recipe for Treating High Cholesterol</u>

Recipe: Cholesterol-Lowering Salad
Ingredients:

FOR THE SALAD

- 2 cups mixed leafy greens
- 1 cup cherry tomatoes
- 1/2 cucumber
- 1/2 red bell pepper
- 1/4 red onion,
- 1/4 cup cooked quinoa or brown rice
- 1/4 cup cooked lean protein
- 1/4 avocado
- Two tablespoons chopped walnuts or almonds

- Fresh herbs (such as parsley, cilantro, or basil) for garnish

FOR THE DRESSING

- 2 tbsp extra-virgin olive oil
- 1 tbsp balsamic vinegar or lemon juice
- 1 tsp Dijon mustard
- One clove of garlic, minced
- Salt and black pepper, to taste

Instructions:

- Wash and chop all the vegetables in a large bowl and mix with quinoa and lean protein.
- Prepare dressing in another bowl by mixing the given quantity.
- Drizzle the sauce over the salad and mix well.
- You can set the spices according to your preference.

HIVES

An allergic reaction usually caused by medications or food is known as hives. However, viruses, dry chemicals, detergents, and stress can also cause this allergy. **The common symptoms of hives are local red-colored bumps, burning, itching, and swelling beneath the skin.** Hives can be acute and chronic. Critical condition is self-limiting, but chronic is severe and requires proper medications.

NATURAL REMEDIES

1. **Oats:** You can take a cheesecloth/sock to wrap the oat around the faucet opening. Take a bath with water that runs through the oat.
2. **Licorice-Chamomile Spray:** Combining these two roots with hazel will relieve the inflammation and itching caused by hives. Mix 2 tbsp of licorice tincture, 2 tbsp of chamomile tincture, and ¾ cup of hazel to prepare the spray. Spray this mixture 2-4 times a day on affected skin.
3. **Melissa and Chamomile Oil:** Mix two drops of Melissa and four drops of chamomile oil in a tepid water tub and bathe for smooth skin.
4. **Aloe Vera Gel:** Rub fresh aloe vera on affected skin a few times daily to relieve irritation and burning.
5. **Cold Compress:** You can use a frozen cloth or ice wrapped in a cloth for compression.

<u>Recipe for Treating Hives</u>

Recipe: Rosemary-Comfrey Salve
Ingredients:
- 1 oz dry crumbled rosemary
- 1 oz beeswax
- 1 oz dry comfrey
- 1 cup olive oil

Instructions:

- Combine olive oil, rosemary, and comfrey in a slow cooker.
- Use the lowest heat setting, cover, and steep herbs for 3-5 hours. Turn off the heat, and let the infused oil cool.
- Simmer water in a double boiler and reduce to low heat.
- Place the cheesecloth on a double boiler and pour in infused oil.
- Squeeze out oil from cheesecloth and discard herbs.
- Add beeswax to infused oil and gently warm over low heat.
- Once beeswax melts, remove it from heat.
- Pour salve into clean jars or tins, and let cool completely before capping.
- Apply dime-size balm to hives with a cotton pad or fingertips 3-4 times daily until hives disappear.

HOT FLASHES

Hot flashes are a symptom of menopause where the upper body feels sudden heat sensations. It starts with abdominal discomfort and chills, then a sudden heat wave passes through the body, and then sweating. Changes in the menopause-associated hormones cause these flashes. Hot flashes usually last for 30 seconds to minutes. **Common symptoms of flashes are high heart rate, headache, nausea, and dizziness.**

NATURAL REMEDIES

1. **Soy:** According to studies, soy can significantly decrease the severity and frequency of hot flashes by up to 11-50%. These plants have a compound like a phytoestrogen that deals with high levels of estrogen that cause hot flashes.
2. **Black Cohosh:** Take one tsp of black cohosh and simmer in hot water for 10-15 minutes. Take this tea three times a day. Take 20mg twice a day if you are taking capsules.
3. **Ground Flax:** Take 1-2 tbsp of ground flaxseed daily for hot flashes.
4. **Sage- Fennel Extract:** Boil one tsp of sage and one tsp of funnel in two cups of water for 5-10 minutes. Strain and consume the section.
5. **Peppermint Oil:** Sniff the oil directly from a bottle, pour a few drops on the tissue, and breathe slowly.
6. **Pumpkin Seed Oil:** You can consume the oil by mixing it with salad dressing, drizzling over bread, or in soap.
7. **Olive Oil Dressing:** Blend ¾ tsp dried oregano, 60 ml red wine vinegar, 60ml extra virgin oil, a pinch of black pepper, and salt. Sprinkle the seasoning on the salad and enjoy.

<u>Recipe for Treating Hot Flashes</u>

Recipe: Lentil Soup
Ingredients:

- 288g dry lentils
- Two celery stalks

- Two diced carrots
- ½ tsp ground cumin
- 411g chopped tomatoes
- Three garlic cloves and one onion
- Two bay leaves
- 1g dry sage
- 946ml vegetable stock
- 28 ml vegetable oil
- Sea salt and black pepper

Instructions:

- Sauté garlic and onion in a pan for 2 minutes.
- Add celery, carrots, and tomato to the pan and sauté for a few minutes.
- After 3-5 minutes, add lentil cumin, bay leaves, sage, stock, pepper and salt and boil.
- Leave the soup on low flame for 15-20 minutes. Decorate the soap with leaves and serve.

IMPOTENCE

Impotence is the inability to maintain or achieve an erection that can lead to satisfying sexual activity. This condition can be psychological due to smoking, diabetes, being overweight, high cholesterol, etc. **Signs of impotence include difficulty achieving or maintaining erections, reduced sexual desire, variability in erection quality, and emotional distress.**

NATURAL REMEDIES

1. **Ginkgo:** A person should take 60-120 mg herb extract every morning for 6 months.
2. **Asian Ginseng:** When using Asian ginseng, it's essential to consider healthcare professionals' instructions and take standardized extracts or supplements. It's crucial to consult with a doctor before use, especially if you're currently taking medication or have any underlying health conditions.
3. **Yohimbe:** A person should take 30-50 mg of yohimbe extract orally. You will see the precise results in 2-3 weeks.
4. **Acupuncture:** Acupuncture is an alternative therapy where thin needles are used to increase the blood flow in specific areas of the body. Some men with erectile dysfunction have reported improvement with acupuncture.
5. **Dietary Changes:** Make a diet plan enriched with fruits, veggies, whole grains, lean proteins, and healthy fats. Foods high in antioxidants, such as berries and nuts, may also help improve blood flow.

Recipe for Treating Impotence

Recipe: Arugula and Beet Salad with Citrus Vinaigrette
Ingredients:

FOR THE SALAD

- 4 cups dry arugula (rocket) leaves

- Two medium beets
- 1/2 cup crumbled feta cheese (optional)
- 1/4 cup walnuts
- 1/4 red onion
- One orange

FOR THE CITRUS VINAIGRETTE

- 3 tbsp extra-virgin olive oil
- 2 tbsp fresh orange juice
- 1 tbsp fresh lemon juice
- 1 tsp honey or maple syrup
- Salt and pepper to taste

Instructions:

- Whisk all the ingredients of citrus vinaigrette in a bowl and set aside.
- Roost the beets in the oven until they become tender.
- Slice all the salad ingredients in a large bowl, including beets.
- Mix the citrus vinaigrette with sliced ingredients, and your salad is ready.

INCONTINENCE

Incontinence refers to the inability to control the discharge of urine or feces from the body. **Symptoms encompass involuntary urine or fecal leakage.** Its causing factors include issues with the muscles in the bladder or rectum, certain medical conditions, hormonal changes, nerve damage, and UTIs.

NATURAL REMEDIES

1. **Kegel Exercises:** Place your pelvic floor muscles on a soft pad by laying flat on your back. Contract your muscles for 5 sec and relax. Repeat the process ten times for about a month. You will observe a difference.
2. **Saw Palmetto:** This herb is sometimes used to support prostate health in men and may have some benefits for urinary symptoms.
3. **Gosha-jinki-gan:** It is a traditional Japanese herbal formula known to enhance bladder control and reduce urinary urgency.
4. **Horsetail:** Horsetail is known for its diuretic properties. It might help with fluid retention and alleviate some incontinence symptoms.
5. **Lavender:** Lavender oil's calming effects help with managing stress-related incontinence and promoting relaxation.
6. **Cranberry Tea:** Cranberry is known for its potential to support urinary tract health and might help prevent urinary tract infections, which can exacerbate incontinence symptoms.

Recipe: Bladder Health Smoothie

Ingredients:

- 1 cup water or unsweetened almond milk
- 1/2 cup fresh or frozen blueberries
- 1/2 cup fresh pineapple chunks
- 1 medium banana
- 1/2 cucumber, peeled and sliced
- One small carrot, peeled and chopped
- 1 tbsp chia seeds
- 1 tbsp flax seeds
- 1/2 cup plain Greek yogurt (optional)
- A handful of spinach or kale leaves
- Ice cubes (optional)

Instructions:

- Put all the ingredients in a blender, along with almond milk or water.
- Blend to get a smooth and creamy texture.
- If desired, add some ice cubes.
- Once blended, enjoy.

INGROWN HAIRS

Ingrown hairs/pseudofolliculitis occur when hair grows sideways into the skin or curls back instead of coming out from the hair follicle. **These hairs can cause inflammation or painful bumps and seem unpleasant.** These hairs are commonly a result of shaving, waxing, or plucking, and they can be more prevalent in areas with coarse or curly hair.

NATURAL REMEDIES

1. **Aspirin-Honey Mask:** Take one tsp warm oil/water and mix with one tsp of honey and three crushed aspirin tablets and mix well. Apply the mask for 10 minutes and then wash.
2. **Sugar Scrub:** Add a cup of sugar into half a cup of coconut oil and a few drops of essential oil. Scrub this paste on your skin with a soft hand. After a few minutes of scrubbing, wash the skin and moisturize.
3. **Oatmeal Paste:** Mix the same amount of oatmeal and baking soda with water to paste. Apply it to the affected area. Leave the paste for 10-20 minutes, and then rinse off.
4. **Apple Cider Vinegar:** Blend equivalent water and apple cider vinegar and put the mixture on the impacted spot using a cotton ball.
5. **Tea Tree Oil:** Combine a few drops of tea tree and a carrier oil and apply using a cotton ball.
6. **Witch Hazel:** Apply with a cotton pad and gently dab it onto the ingrown hair bumps.

Recipe: Soothing Ingrown Hair Treatment Mask

Ingredients:

- 1 tbsp plain yogurt
- 1 tbsp raw honey
- 1 tsp oat flour
- 2-3 drops lavender essential oil (optional)

Instruction:

- Mix all the ingredients to make a paste.
- Wash your skin well before applying the mask.
- Apply the mask with a clean brush. Avoid applying on bruised or cut skin.
- Leave the mask for 10-20 minutes and rinse with warm water.

INSECT BITES AND STINGS

Insects' bites cause a bit of swelling and uncomfortable itching. Common insects like fleas, mosquitos, ants, gnats, etc. are non-poisonous. However, their bites release secretions inside our bodies that cause allergic reactions. **This reaction involves redness, swelling, itching, pain, and local skin reactions.**

NATURAL REMEDIES

1. **Basil-Mullein Salve:** Blend one tbsp of honey, one tsp of mullein, and one tbsp of basil and apply the paste on insect bites for relaxation. You can store this paste in the refrigerator for up to 2 days.
2. **Essential Oils:** Mix one part of **Helichrysum oil** with four parts of **lavender oil**. Apply one drop of this mixture on insect bites 3-4 times daily. It will help with the itching and inflammation. Make a paste of **baking soda in lavender oil** and apply for stings. Baking soda will minimize the inflammation and itching by neutralizing the insect toxins.
3. **Oatmeal Bath:** Place the oatmeal in a cheesecloth and tie the cloth around the faucet. The water in the bathtub will run through the oatmeal. Take a bath and relax. You can directly apply the oatmeal paste on the affected area to limit swelling and irritation.
4. **Witch Hazel:** Apply witch hazel directly on the bite area to relieve irritation and inflammation and soothe skin.
5. **Activated Charcoal:** Take activated charcoal powder from capsules. Mix the powder with water or a few essential or coconut oil drops. Apply the paste on insect bites. This paste will work within 30 minutes only.
6. **Ice Compress:** Applying ice on the sting will relieve pain and prevent inflammation and venom-spread.

Recipe: Peppermint-Plantain Balm for Insect Bites and Stings

Ingredients:

- 2 tbsp dried plantain leaves
- 1/4 cup coconut oil
- 1 tbsp beeswax pellets
- Ten drops peppermint essential oil
- Small glass jar or tin for storage

Instructions:

- Add leaves and coconut oil to a cooker and steep for 3-5 hours on low flame.
- After the oil cools down, strain the leaves from the oil.
- Melt beeswax pellets in a separate container.
- Mix infused oil with melted beeswax.
- Add peppermint oil to the mixture and stir well
- Pour mixture into a clean jar or tin and allow to cool down.
- The mixture will solidify into balm after cooling down.
- Apply the cream on the affected area for relief.

INSOMNIA

A condition of sleeplessness where a person is unable to get good sleep has problems falling asleep or doesn't get enough sleep. There are various reasons for insomnia, like depression, disease, poor environment/ lifestyle/ diet/ physical & mental health, and many more. **The condition can cause extreme anxiety, lack of concentration, fatigue, delayed response, etc.**

NATURAL REMEDIES

1. **Chamomile:** Add 1 tsp of dried chamomile flowers in two cups of boiling water. Boil water for 5 minutes till one cup of water remains. Strain the water and add 1-2 tsp of honey for sweetness. Drink the tea 30-45 minutes before sleep.

2. **Lavender Oil:** There are various ways to use this oil, like:
   - Sniffing
   - Spraying the oil and water mixture on your pillow and sheet
   - Adding a few drops in a vaporizer for 30 minutes

3. **Valerian:** Steep 1 tsp of dried valerian roots in a cup of water for 5-10 minutes. Strain and drink the water 1-2 hours before sleep time.

4. **Kava:** The Piper methysticum roots are used to make kava. Take this drink 2-3 times a day for insomnia.

5. **Passionflower and Linden Elixir**
   - Mix half a cup of raw honey and 1.5 cups of brandy in a jar to prepare the tonic.
   - Then add ¾ cup of dried linden, ¾ cup of dried passionflower, and one lemon zest to the above mixture.

- Stir well and store the tonic in a sterilized bottle.
- Take one tsp of elixir with plain brandy or tea.

6. **Peppermint and Dandelion Tea:** Take 5-10 dandelion leaves, 5-10 peppermint leaves, and 2-inches fresh ginger slices. Steep these ingredients in a cup of hot water for 5 minutes. Strain the water and add honey for sweetness if desired. Take this tea half an hour before the sleep time.

<u>Recipe for Treating Insomnia</u>

Recipe: Sleep Time Balm

Ingredients:
- 1/4 cup coconut oil (solid)
- 1 tbsp beeswax pellets
- 10 drops of lavender essential oil
- Five drops of cedarwood essential oil
- Five drops of bergamot essential oil
- Small glass jar or tin for storage

Instructions:
- Melt the beeswax and coconut oil.
- Cool down the mixture slightly.
- Add the given amount of lavender, cedarwood, and bergamot oils to the mixture. Stir well.
- Pour the mixture and container and allow to cool down till it becomes solid.
- Take a small amount of balm and massage on your neck, soles, temples, and wrist before bedtime.

IRRITABLE BOWEL SYNDROME (IBS)

IBS is a common gastrointestinal disorder. **It is characterized by recurring abdominal pain, discomfort, and alteration in bowel habits, such as Diarrhea , constipation, or both.** The exact reason for IBS is unclear, but factors like sensitive intestines, diet, stress, and gut-brain interactions are believed to play a role. Management of IBS involves dietary modifications, stress reduction, medications, lifestyle changes, etc.

NATURAL REMEDIES

1. **Agrimony:** Steep 1-2 teaspoons of dried agrimony and leave in hot water for 10-15 minutes to make the tea.
2. **Artichoke:** Following the manufacturer's recommendations, you can consume artichoke as a cooked vegetable or take artichoke extract supplements.
3. **Peppermint:** Adults can take 0.2-0.4 ml of peppermint oil three times a day.
4. **Turmeric:** According to studies, turmeric can reduce the IBS symptoms by up to 60%. You can use turmeric in different ways, like milk, vegetable oil, eggs, tea, etc.
5. **Slippery Elm:** Mix 1-2 tsp of its powder with water to create a soothing drink. Consume it 1-3 times a day.

6. **Chamomile:** Steep 1-2 tsp of dried chamomile flowers in hot water for 10-15 minutes. Drink chamomile tea 2-3 times a day.

7. **Fennel:** Chew on fennel and anise seeds after meals or prepare fennel tea by steeping 1-2 teaspoons of crushed fennel seeds in hot water.

Recipe for Treating Irritable Bowel Syndrome (IBS)

Recipe: Gut-Soothing Salad

Ingredients:
- 2 cups mixed leafy greens (spinach, kale, or lettuce)
- 1/2 cup cooked quinoa
- 1/2 cup cooked and cooled lean protein (chicken, turkey)
- 1/2 cup grated carrots
- 1/2 cup cucumber, diced
- 1/4 cup cooked and cooled low-FODMAP vegetables (like zucchini bell peppers)
- 2 tbsp sliced almonds
- 2 tbsp extra-virgin olive oil
- 1 tbsp lemon juice
- 1 tsp fresh grated ginger
- Salt and pepper to taste

Instructions:
- Wash and cut the green vegetables in a bowl.
- Add cooked lean protein, carrots, diced cucumber, and cooled low-FODMAP and quinoa into the salad.
- Make the almond golden brown in a pan for garnishing.
- Add another bowl to make the sauce. Mix well with oil, salt, pepper, lemon juice, and grated ginger.
- Mix the sauce with vegetables and serve.

JET LAG

If you travel quickly across several time zones, dealing with temporary sleep problems is common - this sleep disorder is known as jet lag. Most of us don't know that our body has an internal clock that signals the body when to wake up and when to sleep. This internal clock only synced with your original time zone. **Several mood changes, constipation, Diarrhea , inability to function correctly, and daytime fatigue are common signs of jet lag.**

NATURAL REMEDIES

1. **Essential Oils:** You can take a bath at bedtime with a sprinkling of lavender essential oil or sniff it. Or you can use peppermint oil.

2. **Eat Lightly:** If you want to tackle jet lag effortlessly, eat lightly the day before and the day after you travel. Take food with low carbohydrates and high protein.

3. **Avoid Eating While Flying:** Don't eat heavy meals while flying. Just eat vegetables, fruit, and protein. You can order fruit salad or green salad as your special meal.

4. **Stay Hydrated:** Drink a lot of water before the flight and even during the flight. Take a big glass of water and drink it every hour.

5. **Ginger:** Take ginger candies with you as it is best to treat your airsickness and prevent the constipation that sometimes occurs due to jet lag.

JOCK ITCH

This skin condition is caused by fungal infection. Jock itch mainly occurs as an itchy rash in moist and warm areas of your body, like the inner thighs. Most people know jock itch with the name of tinea cruris, and it looks ring-shaped. **Symptoms of this skin condition include itchiness, scaly skin, a rash that looks like a ring shape, and small blisters.**

NATURAL REMEDIES

1. **Garlic Oil:** Make garlic oil to treat jock itch. Applying infused garlic oil with a pungent smell soothes your irritated skin and kills fungus.

2. **Apple Cider Vinegar:** Take a spritz bottle and combine equal water and apple cider vinegar. Place this in the refrigerator. Apply it directly to the inflamed skin.

3. **Tea Tree Oil:** Add 3-5 drops of tea tree oil in a carrier oil and apply to your affected area. It will give you a soothing feeling and heal the symptoms of jock itch.

KIDNEY STONES

This kidney condition is also known as calculi or urolithiasis. Kidney stones are a form of hard deposits made of minerals and salts. The causes of this condition vary from person to person. The most common conditions are excess body weight, different medical conditions, medications, and supplements. **Severe pain below the ribs, burning sensation, pain fluctuating in intensity, red, pink, or brown urine, cloudy-smelling urine, and urinating more often are the common signs of kidney stones.**

NATURAL REMEDIES

1. **Drink More Water:** Upping your water intake can help you speed up passing kidney stones. Drink up to 2-3 liters of water to prevent kidney stones.

2. **Apple Cider Vinegar:** Take 7-8 ounces of water and add 2 tbsp of apple cider vinegar. Drinking this eases pain caused by stones and reduces the formation of kidney stones.

3. **Hydrangea Roots:** Take 325 mg of each (9 capsules) daily until you feel your pain is over. Drink a lot of water, at least 8 ounces each day.

4. **Cut Back on Salt:** If you are facing kidney problems, you must avoid food with high doses of sodium because it increases calcium excretion through urine.

KNEE PAIN

Different reasons like injury can cause knee pain, medical conditions like gout, arthritis, or ruptured ligament. **The most noticeable signs of knee pain are stiffness, swelling, instability, redness, or crunching noises.**

NATURAL REMEDIES

1. **Apple Cider Vinegar:** Take two tbsp of apple cider vinegar in one glass of water; that will help relieve joint pain.
2. **Willow Bark:** Willow Bark can be taken in tea form, powdered form, or natural pills also available. Take one dose of natural drugs daily to treat knee pain.
3. **Comfrey:** It is a clinically proven natural pain reliever. You can make oil or salve using comfrey leaves. It is the best traditional natural treatment that reduces painful inflammation and soothes skin.

Note: Comfrey is for external use only.

LACTOSE INTOLERANCE

Stomach intolerance is an ailment in which the stomach cannot produce lactose-digesting enzymes. Lactose is not digested in this condition. The causes may be genetic or not. Some people may have a little glass of milk without experiencing symptoms, but others may be unable to have milk in their tea or coffee. They could include **stomach cramps and pain, stomach rumbling, Diarrhea, and bloating stomach.** The degree and timing of your symptoms are determined by the lactose amount you have consumed.

NATURAL REMEDIES

1. **Cocoa Powder:** According to research, cocoa powder and sugar, or chocolate powders, may help the body digest lactose by decreasing the rate at which the stomach empties; the slower the emptying process, the less lactose enters your system at once.
2. **Chocolate Milk:** Chocolate milk contains the same amount of calcium as regular milk, and you may tolerate flavored milk better than plain milk.
3. **Ginger:** Ginger is highly beneficial in treating gastrointestinal problems caused by lactose intolerance or digestion since it efficiently reduces nausea and abdominal gas. You can use it as ginger tea by adding ginger in warm water. Use it daily for better results.
4. **Chamomile:** Chamomile neutralizes stomach acid and aids in bloating reduction. Another advantage is that it encourages relaxation. To brew tea, combine two teaspoons of dried chamomile flowers with a cup of hot water. Drink it several times every day.
5. **Hard Cheese:** If you find yourself tempted to the cheese section of your supermarket, choose hard cheeses such as Swiss, cheddar, and Colby: the harder the cheese, the lower the lactose level.

6. **Soy Milk:** Soya milk is not technically a dairy product. Still, it is often used as a replacement for milk for persons with lactose intolerance or dairy allergies or for vegans who avoid all animal products.

LEG SWELLING

Peripheral edema is leg swelling induced by fluid retention in leg tissues. An issue with the venous circulation system, the lymphatic system, or the kidneys can all cause it. **A part of your body is more significant than it was the day before, the skin surrounding the swelling area appears stretched and glossy, walking becomes difficult if your legs, ankles, or feet swell, and a feeling of fullness or tightness in your swollen body part and mild soreness or an achy sensation in the affected area** are the most prominent symptoms of leg swelling.

NATURAL REMEDIES

1. **Lepas Application:** Lepas are Ayurvedic pastes applied to our bodies, and some assist in reducing swollen legs. A semisolid paste from ginger herbs and deodar (cedar) can help reduce foot swelling.
2. **Essential Oils:** Essential oils such as peppermint, lavender, marjoram, and chamomile can relieve swelling. They are considered to be effective in leg swelling by many researchers.
3. **Ayurvedic Herbs:** Arjuna, punarnava, and adraka (ginger) can be used in powders, pastes, decoctions, juices, and herbal wines in doses prescribed by an Ayurvedic physician.
4. **Watermelon:** Watermelon is an excellent diuretic since it contains 92% water and encourages urination. Watermelons are natural diuretics which assist in minimizing water retention and edema in the foot. In the blazing heat, stock up on watermelons to keep your feet healthy.
5. **Coriander Seeds:** Add 2 to 3 tablespoons of coriander seeds to a cup of water and boil until the quantity is reduced by half. Then strain the solution, let it cool somewhat, and enjoy. Repeat twice daily.
6. **Epsom Salt Bath:** Magnesium sulfate, often known as Epsom Salt, can assist in reducing muscle spasms, inflammation, and swelling, the latter two of which contribute to symptomatic alleviation of edema. Soak your legs in warm water for at least 20 minutes.

LICE INFECTION

The parasitic skin invasion caused by tiny wingless insects is known as lice infestation. Close person-to-person contact is the most common way lice spread. Itching is common in those who have lice. The symptoms of lice people feel are **itching, a tickling feeling, sores on the neck and shoulder, and bite marks.** Lice live on the human head, body, and pubic area and feed on human blood.

NATURAL REMEDIES

1. **Lice Lambaster Liquid:** This oil suffocates lice, eliminating them without the use of harsh chemicals that can irritate the scalp.

2. **Apple Cider Vinegar:** If over-the-counter lice treatments are unavailable or too harsh for your skin, rinse your hair with full-strength apple cider and let it dry naturally. It kills the adult lice and dissolves the eggs. The adhesive that adheres the eggs to the hair shaft is taken. Now, wash your hair with shampoo and apply olive oil on it. The olive oil will make any leftover lice or eggs visible; you must then remove them with a comb and rewash your hair. Repeat every day until the lice are gone.

3. **Lice Repellent:** Pour distilled water into a 16-ounce glass spray bottle. You can make lice repellent by following our instructions. Mix 30 drops of tea tree, five drops of essential oil, and ten drops of oil of your choice, such as lavender, thyme, and cinnamon. Fill hazel in the bottle. Shake lightly before spraying over the scalp and back of the neck.

Recipe for Treating Lice Repellent

Recipe: Lice Lambaster Liquid

Ingredients:
- Two tablespoons black walnut–infused oil
- Two tablespoons rosemary-infused oil
- Two tablespoons sage-infused oil
- Two tablespoons fennel-infused oil

Instructions:
- Mix black walnut-infused oil, sage-infused oil, and rosemary-infused oil.
- Transfer it to the bottle. Tighten the bottle's lid and label it with the name of the formula and the date it was created.
- Massage a generous amount of oil into the scalp. Cover with a shower cap and leave for 30 minutes before combing out the lice with a lice comb.

MENOPAUSE

The time of stopping your menstrual cycle is called menopause. Menopause can occur in your 40s or 50s, the average age; anything between 41 and 49 is considered normal. **The symptoms include irregular periods, night sweats or hot flashes, vaginal dryness, chills, sleeping problems, mood swings, weight gain, skin changes, loss of breast fullness, and painful sex.**

NATURAL REMEDIES

1. **Black Cohosh:** For black cohosh tincture, 2 to 4 ml diluted in water or tea once to thrice a day can be used for hot flashes. You can take one or two 40-mg capsules or extract (standardized to 2.5% triterpene glycosides) twice daily to ward against menopausal symptoms.

2. **Red Clover :** Red clover, a member of the legume family (which also includes peas and beans), is found to be suitable for treating menopause. Red clover extracts are advertised as a treatment for hot flashes and other menopause symptoms.

3. **Saged Iced Tea:** In 8 oz of water, steep 1 tbsp of the fresh or dried herb for 5 to 10 minutes. Refine, calm, and sip.

4. **Kava:** Multiple studies have demonstrated that kava considerably lowers anxiety and is effective for menopause symptoms; it can alleviate anxiety and sleep problems.

5. **Isoflavones :** According to research, 20-60 mg/day or 34-76 mg isoflavone can lessen hot flashes. Additionally, meals including soy, leafy dark greens, and walnuts are high in calcium and magnesium, which are suitable for the bones—according to studies, consuming more soy isoflavones after menopause reduces bone loss.

<u>Recipe for Treating Menopause</u>

Recipe: Almond Pancakes - Good for Energy Stabilizing

Ingredients:

- 75g oats
- 60g almond flour
- 1 tbsp ground flaxseeds
- ½ tsp cinnamon
- ½ tsp sea salt
- 1 tsp baking powder
- 175ml unsweetened almond milk (or milk of your choice)
- ½ tsp baking soda
- Two eggs
- Coconut oil for frying
- 1 tsp pure vanilla extract

TOPPING INGREDIENTS

- 1 tbsp pure maple syrup
- 50g blueberries
- A drizzle of almond butter and your favorite raw seeds

Instructions:

- Mix the eggs, milk, and vanilla to the blender.
- Heat the saucepan for 5 minutes and add in coconut oil.
- When the oil melts, pour pancakes about three inches into the pan.
- After three to four minutes, when the pancakes turn golden and small holes appear on the uncooked side, flip and cook for another two to three minutes.

MENSTRUAL CRAMPS

Menstrual cramps are common sharp pains in the lower abdomen during the menstrual cycle days. Dysmenorrhea is the term doctors use to describe period pain since it may be severe. **The symptoms include cramping pain in the lower abdomen, continuous aches, nausea, loose stools, headache, and dizziness.**

NATURAL REMEDIES

1. **Ginger:** When eaten three times daily during the menstrual cycle, an eighth of a teaspoon of ginger powder relieves cramps and lessens bleeding.

2. **Take Massage:** A 20-minute massage can be helpful. The hands of the massage therapist go over your abdomen, side, and back while he presses specific points as you go through your menstrual cycle. For an aromatherapy-style acupressure, using essential oils may have further advantages.

3. **Chamomile Tea:** The antispasmodic effects of chamomile tea help ease the excruciating cramps related to menstrual cycles. Additionally, the tea impacts on dopamine and serotonin are modulated, helping to neutralize or at least lessen the effects of depressive symptoms.

4. **Cinnamon:** Consume 2-3 cups of cinnamon tea one to two days before starting periods to avoid cramps. Drink it 2-3 times on the 1st day of your period to relieve period pain.

5. **French Maritime Pine Bark Extract:** During your cycle, consume 60 mg of French maritime pine bark extract daily.

6. **Dill:** Early studies indicate that consuming dill for three days at the onset of pain helps women with menstrual cramps feel less pain. Take 1,000 mg of dill five days before your period and continue for five days.

Recipes for Treating Menstrual Cramps

Recipe 1: Sweet Spice Tea

Ingredients:

- 2 cups (475 ml) water
- Two teaspoons (4 g) aniseeds
- One teaspoon (2 g) celery seeds
- One tablespoon (2 g)
- Dried peppermint leaves
- ¼ teaspoon saffron
- Honey or stevia (optional)

Instructions:

- Boil the water. Combine the anise, celery, peppermint, and saffron in a teapot or dish. Boiling water should be added.
- For 15 to 20 minutes, let the tea steep. Strain. If desired, add sweetness to taste.

Recipe 2: Olive-Topia Tapenade

Ingredients:

- ¼ cup (25 g) pitted black olives
- Minced fresh garlic
- Chopped finely 1½ teaspoons (5 g)
- Olive oil
- Pinch of sea salt Small loaf of crusty French bread

Instructions:

- Heated the oven to 350°F
- The garlic and chopped olives should be mixed in a small basin.
- Add just enough olive oil to help the mixture come together.
- Add a dash of sea salt and stir. Slice the bread into 2.5 cm pieces.
- Apply the tapenade and heat the oven.
- Spread the tapenade on top and reheat in the oven for a little while.

MORNING SICKNESS

Morning sickness is very common during pregnancy. In the first trimester, about 8 out of 10 women are affected by morning sickness. Its symptoms decrease at the start of the 2nd trimester commonly. **The symptoms include heartburn, motion sickness, hunger pangs, and feeling like something is stuck in the throat.**

NATURAL REMEDIES

1. **Apple Cider Vinegar:** A pleasant equilibrium of stomach acids can be achieved in the morning by drinking an apple cider vinegar tonic.
2. **Peppermint Oil:** An upset stomach can be calmed by taking peppermint as capsules or drinking it in tea.
3. **Ginger:** Natural nausea relief comes from ginger. It has anti-inflammatory qualities that aid in enhancing digestion.
4. **Cinnamon Bark:** The cinnamon tree produces cinnamon bark, frequently suggested as a chemotherapy nausea remedy. Cinnamon helps ease muscle tension, calm the stomach, and promote digestion.

Recipes for Treating Morning Sickness

Recipe 1: Chamomile-Ginger Tea
Ingredients:

- 1 cup boiling water
- One teaspoon dried chamomile
- One teaspoon chopped fresh ginger root

Instructions:

- In a big mug, pour the boiling water. Then, cover the mug and let the tea steep for 10 minutes with the chamomile and ginger.
- Breathe in the steam, unwind, and sip the tea leisurely. Repeat every day, up to four times.

Recipe 2: Comforting Potato-Cauli Mash
Ingredients:

- Two boiled potatoes
- Peeled one garlic clove
- Minced ½ head cauliflower

- Steamed until easily pierced with a fork
- Freshly ground black pepper

Instructions:
- In a medium bowl, mash the warm potatoes.
- Add the minced garlic and stir.
- Mash the warm cauliflower in a different bowl.
- Combine cauliflower and potatoes.
- Include the pepper, then consume while still heated.

MOTION SICKNESS

Motion sickness, brought on by a moving vehicle, is characterized by **nausea, dizziness, headaches, increased salivation, anxiety, cold sweat, and tiredness.**

NATURAL REMEDIES

1. **Candied Ginger:** It's convenient to ingest candied ginger, making it a great travel companion. The dosage is 1 pound for motion sickness.
2. **Peppermint:** Both peppermint (Mentha piperata) tincture and essential oil may be good to keep on hand. The tincture can be ingested as a motion sickness remedy, while the essential oil can be inhaled.
3. **Black Horehound:** Even though black horehound is occasionally used by those who suffer from motion sickness. Black horehound may be detrimental to some Parkinson's patients since it can interact with their meds.
4. **Ginger:** Ginger can be effective for motion sickness. It is commonly used as a slice to stop the symptoms of motion sickness.

Recipe for Treating Motion Sickness

Recipe: Candied Ginger

Ingredients:

- 5 cups water
- 1 pound fresh ginger root peeled and cut into ⅛-inch-thick slices
- 1 pound raw cane sugar

Instructions:

- Take parchment paper and put it on your baking tray.
- Combine water and ginger in a saucepan and cook over medium-high heat.
- Bring the mixture to boil on medium heat.
- Combine sugar and boiled ginger for 20 minutes and stir it continuously on low flame until it crystallizes.
- Use a fork to transfer the crystallized pieces of ginger to the rack.
- Store it after cooling for two weeks in the container.

MUSCLE STRAIN

Muscle strain occurs when a muscle or tendon is too stretched or under excessive pressure. A muscle or tendon can be overstretched and healed with ice and rest. Or a tendon may tear entirely or partially, necessitating surgery. **A muscular strain is characterized by acute pain that worsens when the muscle is contracted, swelling and bruising, loss of strength, and restricted range of motion.**

NATURAL REMEDIES

1. **Juniper Berry:** This essential oil, made from the berries of the common evergreen plant, has an energizing, woodsy-sweet, pine-needle-like scent that boosts energy to increase output and attentiveness.
2. **Raw Onion:** Even though all veggies are necessary for good health, onions are among the best for easing pain. Numerous vitamins and minerals found in raw onions significantly lessen pain.
3. **Epsom Salt:** According to numerous researches, epsom salt is an excellent treatment for muscle stiffness and discomfort.
4. **Cherry Juice:** In a study that was conducted in 2012, researchers concluded that persons with muscle pain who drink cherry juice two times a day face less pain.
5. **Olive Oil:** When massaged into your body, olive oil can aid in reducing a variety of pain and soreness.

Recipe for Treating Muscle Strain

Recipe: Cherry Juice

Ingredients:

- ¼ cup of water
- 1 cup cherries

Instructions:

- Wash the cherries and take out the pits first.
- Add cold water to the fruit (around 14 cups for every cup of cherry) and blend until it is smooth and juicy.
- If you like pulpy, have some. If not, filter the cherry juice to remove the pulp with a fine mesh sieve or nut milk bag.

NAUSEA AND VOMITING

Nausea may or may not lead to vomiting. It has numerous causes, including food or other poisoning, bacterial or viral infections, inner ear problems, intestinal parasites, morning sickness in pregnancy, motion sickness, migraine headache, intoxication, overeating, certain medications, and stress, anxiety, or shock. **Lack of appetite, excessive sweating, repeated rhythmic contractions of abdominal and respiratory muscles, stomach ache and uneasy feeling** in your chest are the symptoms of vomiting and nausea.

NATURAL REMEDIES

1. **Ginger:** Ginger stimulates digestion, causing the stomach to empty faster while soothing and relaxing the entire system.
2. **Cardamom:** Cardamom is especially good for treating stomach trouble. Traditionally, it has been used to treat a wide range of digestive problems, including nausea.
3. **Peppermint Oil:** It is usually best to use peppermint oil instead of peppermint candies. However, sucking on a peppermint candy in a pinch can certainly help nausea.
4. **Rice Water:** Boil rice and strain its water. After it cools, you need to drink water to help soothe your stomach. It's not suggested that you add any sweetener to this remedy, but luckily, rice water does not have much taste and is easy to stay down. This remedy should work within 10-15 minutes after drinking.

<u>Recipe for Treating Nausea and Vomiting</u>

Recipe: Lavender and Peppermint Essential Oil

Ingredients:

- 1 cup sweet almond oil
- 20 drops of lavender essential oil
- 6 drops peppermint essential oil

Instructions:

- Using a funnel, pour the almond oil into a dark-colored glass bottle, and then add the lavender and peppermint essential oils.
- Label and date the bottle.
- Cover and shake the bottle well before each use.
- You can add 1 spoon in the bathtub of warm water and stay in it for 15 minutes.

NECK PAIN

Cervicalgia, often known as neck pain, is discomfort in or near your spine beneath your head. Your cervical spine is another name for your neck. It is a common ailment in the US, as 80% of adults experience it. **The common symptoms people experience in the case of neck pain are stiffness of the neck, headache, sharp pain around the neck area, pain when moving, and numbness.**

NATURAL REMEDIES

1. **Chamomile:** These daisy-like plant constituents can reduce inflammation and block pain signals. Fill a clean sock with a cup of dried chamomile to relieve back discomfort.
2. **Turmeric and Ginger:** Until your discomfort is reduced, consume 1 to 2 g of each spice daily in supplement form.

3. **Devils Claw:** This shrub is available as pills or powder. The effectiveness of this plant in alleviating neck discomfort is the subject of much research. It has already been found to be effective and suggested by many researchers for reducing neck pain.
4. **Camphor Oil:** Camphor oil can ease skin irritability and relieve pain. It can be applied at the point of neck pain.
5. **Lavender:** The treatment of neck and lower back pain now includes the use of massage oils and aromatherapy.

Recipe for Treating Neck Pain

Recipe: Lavender Mint Tea

Ingredients:

- ¼ cup fresh lavender petals
- 1 cup fresh mint leaves
- 4 cups water

Instructions:

- Add mint and lavender to the pot in which you want to make tea.
- Add water to it and heat till boiling.
- Place the mint and lavender in a pot, add water to cover, and heat until the water is boiling.
- After filtering the mint and lavender blossoms from the tea, serve it hot. If you would like, strain the tea and serve it with ice.

NOSE BLEED

Epistaxis, the medical term for nose bleeding, can be brought on by something as easy as blowing your nose hard. This is so because a capillary can easily break through the nose's relatively thin lining. You can be more susceptible to nosebleeds if you do not get enough vitamin C or use aspirin. **The common symptoms of nosebleed are bleeding from either one or both nostrils, a sensation of liquid flow at the back of the throat, and the urge to swallow frequently.**

NATURAL REMEDIES

1. **Lemon:** A cotton swab with a few drops of lemon essential oil should be softly dipped into the nostril. It is thought to be most effective in the case of nosebleeds.
2. **Cayenne Pepper:** As soon as the bleeding begins, take a teaspoon of cayenne pepper, mix it with warm water, and consume. The blood immediately stops.
3. **Nettle Leaf:** Tea made from fresh nettle leaves should be cooled. After that, dab the cotton pad on the nose with the solution. Keep it there until the bleeding stops, about five to ten minutes.
4. **Saline Water:** Use a bowl, add a few drops of saline water, and some water. To moisten the inner lining of the nasal passages, thoroughly combine it and dispense a few drops of the resulting solution into your nose.

5. **Onion Juice:** After dipping the cotton ball in onion juice, place it for three to four minutes in the affected nostril. Another approach is to place a piece of onion under your nose and breathe in the aroma.

6. **Baking Soda:** Spray it in your nostrils three to four times a day by combining 12 tsp of salt and 14 tsp of baking soda in a glass of water. The bleeding will eventually stop.

OBJECT IN EAR

A foreign item in the ear can lead to pain, infection, and hearing loss if it is not removed. Having a foreign object in your ear can cause discomfort, agony, and even mild hearing loss. However, young kids might not be aware of it. **The signs of a foreign body in the ear are ear pain, dizziness or nausea, trouble in hearing, bleeding or itching in the ear, and foul odor coming from your ear.**

NATURAL REMEDIES

1. **Use Alcohol:** Pour warm (not hot) oil or alcohol into the ear. Oil types include mineral, olive, and baby. The bug ought to float away. If you believe your eardrum may be ruptured or if you have ear tubes in situ, avoid using oil.

2. **Use Warm Olive Oil:** By briefly cradling the bottle in your hands, you can warm the oil. Pull the earlobe back and upward for adults and back and downward for children. Put enough oil in the ear to fill the canal using a dropper.

3. **Use Tweezers:** Use tweezers to carefully remove the thing if it is simple to see and hold. Grab the item in the ear with a pair of soft, soap-clean tweezers. To avoid the item from shattering before it completely exits the ear, move carefully and gently.

4. **Earwax :** Typically, earwax has a consistency similar to toothpaste. The majority of the wax is tightly packed inside the ear canal when it is removed with a Q-Tip or other similar tool.

5. **Tilt Your Head:** An object may occasionally be small or free enough to emerge naturally. Tilt your head to the side and utilize gravity to assist you in removing anything that is caught in your ear. To maximize the likelihood of the thing dropping out on its own, gently shake your head.

6. **Flush the Ear with Water:** Foreign things can be flushed out with water, especially if they are little. Before filling a bulb syringe with warm (not hot) water, wash your hands. Insert the syringe, pull your ear up and back, then slowly squeeze water into your ear.

OBJECT IN EYE

Anything that shouldn't be in your eye, such as a speck of dust, a wood chip, a metal shaving, an insect, or a piece of glass, is referred to as a foreign body. Under your eyelid or on the surface of your eye are the typical locations to locate a foreign body. **There are some signs when you know there is something in your eye, which are sharp pain in your eye, red eyes, blurred vision, sensitivity from bright lights, and bleeding into the whites of the eye.**

1. **Wash the Eye:** Washing the eye can remove the object immediately if it is not deeper.
2. **Saline Solution:** Fill a small, shallow container with water or saline solution. Once it is full, submerge your eyes and attempt to remove the object by repeatedly blinking. The thing could become looser by slightly moving the top eyelid away from the eye.
3. **Use Cotton Swab:** Sometimes, you can't locate the object in the eye; it can be hidden in the eye, such as in the eyelid. Grab the eyelid in this case and pull slowly to make it visible at the lower eyelid. You can use a cotton swab for this purpose. Looking down makes it simpler to accomplish and remove from the eye.
4. **Cold Compress:** If your eyes are slightly inflamed after you remove the object, apply a cool, moist compress to ease the irritation. Until your eyes have totally healed, refrain from wearing eye makeup.
5. **Stand in the Shower:** Additionally, while standing in the shower, you can allow warm water to drip from your head and into your eye. Make sure your shower head is on a lower pressure level if you choose this option and that the stream doesn't directly contact your eye.

ORAL THRUSH

A fungal infection of the mouth is called oral thrush. **White patches in the mouth, redness in the throat and mouth, loss or unpleasant taste in the mouth, cracks at the corners of the mouth, and burning sensations are the main signs of oral thrush.**

NATURAL REMEDIES

1. **Tea Tree:** For oral thrush, buy a diluted form of tea tree oil to use as an oral rinse. You can't really dilute it yourself because the oil doesn't mix with water.
2. **Salt Water:** Using salt water to rinse your mouth may help reduce oral thrush symptoms.
3. **Lemon Juice:** Add the juice of half a lemon to one cup of warm or cool water. Use the liquid to rinse your mouth or consume it. Although some people use lemon juice directly to thrush lesions, the acidity of the lemon may burn and irritate the skin.
4. **Clove Oil:** One cup of boiling water and one teaspoon of whole ground cloves should steep for at least 5 minutes. Use it as a mouthwash to treat oral thrush.
5. **Oregano Oil:** One cup of water and two drops of oregano oil are combined. You should swish the mixture around your mouth.
6. **Gentian Violet:** Gentian violet, often referred to as crystal violet or methyl violet 10b, is a kind of antiseptic dye that was utilized in the 19th century to combat germs, fungi, and parasites. You can use a 1% solution. Apply a small amount to a cotton ball or swab before gently dabbing it on the white spots in your mouth to utilize it.

OSTEOPOROSIS

When the quality of the bone structure is destroyed and the density of bone minerals decreases, it results in osteoporosis. At thirty, when most people stop developing new bones, the deterioration process begins. Women suffer a quickening of this process after menopause, but by the age of 70, the rate of loss reaches a plateau for both genders. **However, once osteoporosis has weakened your bones, you could encounter symptoms like back pain brought on by a broken or collapsed vertebra and a reduction of height over time.**

NATURAL REMEDIES

1. **Green Tea:** Green tea-drinking women have a decreased incidence of osteopenia and osteoporosis. You can take one cup of green tea daily for better results.
2. **Evening Primrose Oil:** Older patients with osteoporosis use evening primrose oil together with fish oil and calcium; this combination appears to reduce bone loss and increase bone density. You can directly apply it to the skin to prevent osteoporosis.
3. **Red Clover:** Red clover's isoflavones appear to prevent women from losing bone mass by functioning in the body like weak estrogens.
4. **Soy:** Soy can both stop bone deterioration and boost bone mineral density. Soy can help women before and after menopause by reducing the symptoms of osteoporosis.
5. **Red Sage:** The plant red sage, also known as danshen in Chinese herbal medicine, has been linked to improvements in osteoporosis. They can be used as a supplement in the form of a tablet, powder, or tea, or they can be utilized in cooking.

Recipe for Treating Osteoporosis

Recipe: Bone-Boosting Tahini
Ingredients:
- 2½ cups (360 g) sesame seeds
- ¾ cup olive oil

Instructions:
- The oven should be preheated to 350°F.
- The seeds of sesame should be spread in it and toast for ten minutes.
- Take the seeds out after 15 minutes from the oven.
- Store the prepared seeds for three or more three weeks in an air container.

PIMPLES

Unpleasant skin lumps filled with pus are called pimples. The medical term used for pimples is acne vulgaris. Blackheads, whiteheads, small red spots with yellow pus, skin scarring, and skin crusting are the main symptoms of pimples.

NATURAL REMEDIES

1. **Apple Cider Vinegar:** Combine three parts water and 1 part apple cider vinegar to treat pimples.
2. **Aloe Vera:** Utilize a spoon to scrape the aloe plant's gel. As a moisturizer, apply the gel to clean the skin.
3. **Grapes Cleanser:** Mash 8-10 grapes. Add 2 tbsp of aloe vera gel and 2 drops of vitamin E oil in the mashed grapes. Massage your face with this mixture. After 20 minutes, wash your face.
4. **Yeast and Yogurt Face Mask:** Thin one teaspoon of brewer's yeast with a small amount of plain yogurt to make the mask. Cook and thoroughly apply it to all oiled areas. Leave on for 15 to 20 minutes. Warm water should be used to rinse, followed by cold water to shut the pores.

Recipe for Treating Pimples

Recipe: Healing Clay Poultice

Ingredients:
- Cosmetic clay Water
- One drop of lavender essential oil

Instructions:
- Make a paste by mixing equal parts water and cosmetic clay.
- Only combine the amount you'll use immediately; to treat a pimple, you'll need about 12 tsp.
- Mix extra if you're addressing a bigger area.
- Test a tiny area before using clay; it can irritate skin that is already sensitive. Before combining the paste, you can, if you'd like, add lavender essential oil to the water.

POISON IVY

In reality, the plant known as "poison ivy" causes dermatitis. It is an itchy, red skin condition that can turn inflammatory. When exposed to poison ivy or oak's oily resin, some people react badly, while others do not. **The symptoms of poison ivy rash include itching, redness, swelling, blisters, and difficulty breathing if inhaled the smoke from burning poison ivy.**

NATURAL REMEDIES

1. **Cucumber:** Although it won't cure your poison ivy, it will undoubtedly soothe the rash. Take a sizable cucumber—or many, depending on the size of the area—and slice it. Slices should be applied to the affected region.
2. **Apple Cider Vinegar:** Apple cider vinegar therapy begins to kill the poison. Your rash will disappear much more quickly. To clean the damaged region, apple cider vinegar is also thought to be antimicrobial.

3. **Oatmeal:** Take an oatmeal bath to get rid of itching. When you take an oatmeal bath and soak for at least an hour, things get better.

<u>Recipe for Treating Poison Ivy</u>

Recipe: Clay Poultice Cosmetic Clay

Ingredients:
- Water 1 drop
- Lavender essential oil (optional)

Instructions:
- Combine equal parts cosmetic clay and water to make a paste.
- Mix only as much as you'll use immediately; to treat a pimple, you'll need just 1/2 tsp. If you're treating a larger area, mix more.
- Before using, test on a small area; clay can irritate sensitive skin. If you like, add lavender essential oil to the water before mixing the paste.

PREMENSTRUAL SYNDROME (PMS)

The discomfort a woman feels before the start of her monthly period is typical. It can be difficult. Premenstrual Syndrome starts 1-2 weeks before a woman's period and ends when the women get their menstrual cycle. **Insomnia, headaches, social withdrawal, poor focus, depression, anxiety, mood swings, and food cravings are the most obvious symptoms seen in patients with PMS.**

NATURAL REMEDIES

1. **Black Cohosh Syrup:** This slightly bitter syrup is a convenient alternative to tea, and it lasts for up to 6 months when stored in the refrigerator. Make 2 cups of water with honey.
2. **Rose:** Premenstrual syndrome (PMS) symptoms and stress can be eased by roses' relaxing aroma.
3. **Chaste Berry:** Women's reproductive systems can benefit from the use of the chaste berry. It can be used in the form of tea. Add 1 tablespoon in 4 cups of boiled water to make tea.
4. **Ginkgo Biloba:** According to a study, symptoms were greatly lessened in women who took tablets containing 40 mg of leaf extract thrice daily for a few days during their menstrual cycles.
5. **Fruit Vitex:** Dried, mature chaste berries are employed to make liquid or solid extracts that are put into capsules and tablets. Additionally, vitex is available as a liquid or tea and in blends with other herbs that support hormonal balance.

<u>Recipe for Treating Premenstrual Syndrome (PMS)</u>

Recipe: Dandelion-Ginger Tea

Ingredients:
- 1 cup boiling water
- 1 teaspoon chopped dandelion root

- 1 teaspoon chopped ginger root

Instructions:

- Fill a large cup halfway with boiling water.
- Allow the tea to brew for 10 minutes after adding the roots.
- Relax and drink the tea slowly while inhaling the steam. Repeat up to four times per day.

PSORIASIS

Psoriasis is a skin disease that causes an itchy, scaly rash on the knees, elbows, trunk, and scalp. While stress management can help you prevent breakouts, relaxing herbal therapies can help you reduce itching, pain, redness, and thick, flaky areas of skin. **The most obvious symptoms of psoriasis are dry and cracked skin, itching, cyclic rashes, and small scaling spots.**

NATURAL REMEDIES

1. **Turmeric:** Turmeric facemasks can be used to calm inflammation and promote skin healing.
2. **Oregon Grapes:** Oregon grape/Mahonia aquafolium contains an antibacterial and anti-inflammatory component called berberine. Applying 10% Oregon grape ointment and cream twice daily treat psoriasis symptoms.
3. **Soak in Oats:** Add a cup of oats to a warm bath and soak it for 15 minutes. You can repeat the procedure for better results.
4. **Tea Tree Oil:** Tea tree oil has antiseptic properties that may prevent infection in psoriasis lesions. Dilute tea tree oil with a carrier oil (e.g., coconut oil) in 1:10 drops and apply sparingly to affected areas.
5. **Aloe Vera:** Apply freshly extracted aloe vera gel on the effective area multiple times for quick relief.

<u>Recipe for Treating Psoriasis</u>

Recipe: Licorice Root Spray

Ingredients:

- ¾ cup witch hazel
- ¼ cup licorice root tincture

Instructions:

- In a dark-colored glass bottle with a spray top, combine the ingredients. Shake gently to blend completely.
- Apply where the psoriasis area is present.
- Repeat the process 3-4 times/day.

RASHES

The red, itchy, and inflamed area on the skin is called rashes. The known causing factors of rashes are allergens, fungi, viruses, bacteria, excessive use of skin products, oily skin, and others. **The symptoms of rashes are fluid-filled blisters, redness, inflammation, itching, and dry skin.**

NATURAL REMEDIES

1. **Chickweed:** Applying chickweed poultices directly on rashes will soothe the irritation, inflammation, and itching. This herb is also effective for other skin conditions like minor burns, cuts, eczema, etc. Only use the flowers and leaves of this herb.
2. **Comfrey:** Leaves and flowers of comfrey also contain amazing properties against many skin problems like rashes, burns, scrapes, and insect bites. You can make herb poultice or buy a cream containing comfrey extract.
3. **Sage:** Apply sage oil leaves extract, or take a sage bath for 10-15 minutes to relieve rashes.
4. **Plantain:** Plantain helps relieve swelling and itching of rashes, insect bites, and others by sucking toxins from the skin. Apply leaves, leaves paste, or oil on any rashes.
5. **Calendula:** Apply calendula oil on different rashes to relieve irritation, swelling, and itching multiple times daily. You can also mix the gel with the oil for improved effects.
6. **Aloe Vera Gel:** Apply the gel directly on the rashes or mix it with oils like witch hazel and calendula for improved effects.
7. **Witch Hazel:** Witch hazel soothes itching and swelling caused by various skin problems or mixed with aloe vera gel.
8. **Oatmeal Bath:** Oatmeal soothes skin irritation caused by rashes, insect bites, poison ivy, sunburns, hives, etc. Take an oatmeal bath by filtering water through it.

Recipe for Treating Rashes

Recipe: Rash Relief Cream

Ingredients:

- 1/4 cup of coconut oil
- 2 tablespoons of aloe vera gel
- 10 drops of lavender oil
- 5 drops of tea tree oil (optional)
- 1 tablespoon of beeswax pellets

Instructions:

- Melt coconut oil and beeswax in a double-boiler or medium flame. Gently mix both ingredients.
- Remove the bowl and let it cool slightly.
- Once the mixture has cooled slightly, add essential oils and aloe gel and mix.
- Pour the cream into a sanitized jar and let it cool down. Apply this cream a few times a day on rashes.

RESTLESS LEGS SYNDROME

It's a neurological disorder that causes a tempting urge to move the legs due to irritated sensations. **The signs of RLS are creeping, itching, throbbing, and tingling sensations in the legs.** It can be related to genetic factors, iron deficiency, certain medical conditions, medications, and pregnancy.

NATURAL REMEDIES

1. **Lavender Oil:** Massage lavender oil on the legs or make an oil spray by mixing it with magnesium and peppermint oil.
2. **Peppermint Oil:** Peppermint oil relaxes muscles, cramps, and pain, while its aroma gives calming effects. You can massage your legs with this oil or add it to your bath water.
3. **Valerian Root:** Valerian roots show clear results in calming the legs and improving sleep. You can consume 800 mg of herbs/per day through tea.
4. **Passionflower:** It can be used in the form of tea. Add one tablespoon of dried herb to a cup. 8 ounces of boiling water should be poured over the herb. You should then cover the cup with a small plate or lid and let it steep for 20 to 30 minutes. Remove the herbs, then pour 4 ounces up to four times daily.
5. **Magnesium:** Magnesium minimizes the symptoms of restless legs syndrome. You can take magnesium supplements or add magnesium-rich food to your diet.
6. **Hot and Cold Compress:** Applying warm or cold packs on your legs or taking a bath can temporarily relieve discomfort and improve blood flow.

Recipe for Treating Restless Legs Syndrome

Recipe: Soothing Herbal Tea

Ingredients:

- 1 tsp of dried valerian root
- 1 tsp of dried passionflower
- 1 tsp of dried chamomile flowers
- 1 tsp of dried lemon balm
- 1 tsp of dried skullcap
- 1 cup of hot water
- Honey (optional, for sweetness)

Instructions:

- Take two cups of water and boil.
- Add all the herbs in boiling water on low flame for 10-15 minutes until water remains half.
- Strain the tea and add honey if required.
- Take a cup of this herbal tea 30-60 minutes before sleep.
- Make sure to consult a specialist before trying this tea.

SHIN SPLINTS

Soreness and pain associated with shin bone are called shin splints. The pain is usually in, behind, or around the shin bone. **This condition is characterized by aching, inner inflammation, and pain that might stop when resting.** The common causes of shin splints are running barefoot or with hard shoes, sudden intensive exercise, running on rough surfaces, dancing, and jumping.

NATURAL REMEDIES

1. **Ice Compress:** Apply an ice pack on your affected leg for 10-20 minutes to treat pain and swelling. Ice decreases the blood flow in particular areas that alleviate pain.

2. **Essential Oil Bath:** Adding a few drops of this oil in a warm water tub will calm your spine pain. Add 1-2 tsp of lavender oil in water and soak your body for 10-20 minutes.

3. **Oil Massage:** To massage the affected area, use essential oils like lavender, marjoram, peppermint, rosemary, etc. These oils will work against pain and swelling by increasing blood flow.

4. **Ginger Roots:** Take 1-2 inches of ginger roots. Use cheesecloth to soak the roots in a warm water tub for 10-15 minutes. Take a bath with ginger water a few times daily.

5. **Cayenne Patches:** Prepare cayenne patches through its paste in water and apply on the affected leg two times daily.

6. **Turmeric:** Make turmeric paste in water, apply on the affected area for 15-20 minutes and rinse with tepid water. This paste will minimize swelling and muscle pain.

<u>Recipe for Treating Shin Splints</u>

Recipe: Soothing Muscle Relief Cream
Ingredients:
- 1/4 cup of coconut oil
- 2 tbsp of shea butter
- 10 drops of peppermint oil
- 10 drops of eucalyptus oil
- 5 drops of lavender oil
- 1 tbsp of beeswax pellets

Instructions:
- Melt coconut oil, beeswax pellets, and shea butter in a double broiler and mix well.
- After the ingredients are mixed properly, let the mixture slightly cool.
- Add the given number of essential oils to the mixture and mix well.
- Transfer the cream to a sterilized jar and let it solidify.
- Gently massage the cream on the pain area twice a day.

SHOULDER PAIN

Any shoulder joint or tendon issue results in sharp, burning shoulder pain. Any injury, joint dislocation, pressure, trapped rotator cuff tendon under bone, fracture, rotator cuff tear, etc. can cause this pain. **The symptoms of shoulder pain can be slow or no arm movement, inflammation, stabbing pain, stiffness, etc. The symptoms can vary based on the pain caused.**

NATURAL REMEDIES

1. **Blue Vervain:** Take dried herbal leaves to make tea or use tinctures.
2. **Turmeric:** Consume turmeric tea thrice daily for joint pain. Add a tsp of ground turmeric in a cup of boiling water, simmer for 10 minutes, strain, and sweeten with honey or lemon to taste.
3. **Essential Oils:** You can massage your affected area with wintergreen, eucalyptus, lavender, chamomile, peppermint, rosemary, or other essential oils.
4. **Willow Bark:** Steep 1 to 2 tsp of dried willow bark in a cup of hot water for 10-15 minutes, then strain and drink up to three times daily. Willow bark contains natural compounds similar to aspirin, which may help alleviate pain and inflammation.
5. **Cold Compress:** Cold compression is effective for instant pain relief and inflammation reduction. Use an ice pack or a cold cloth to compress the shoulder for 10-15 minutes a few times daily.

Recipe for Treating Shoulder Pain

Recipe: Homemade Arnica Gel
Ingredients:
- 1/2 cup of carrier oil
- 1/4 cup of dried arnica flowers
- 2 tbsp of beeswax

Instructions:
- First, make arnica-infused oil.
- Add dried arnica flowers in a dry, clean jar to make the oil.
- Completely submerge the flowers in a carrier oil.
- Close the jar tightly and put it in a dark place for 2-4 weeks. Shake the jar daily.
- After 2-4 weeks, strain the flowers from the oil, and your arnica-infused oil is ready.
- Add arnica-infused oil and beeswax in a double boiler and melt on medium flame.
- Mix them well and place them in a clean jar. Let the mixture cool and solidify. Your arnica gel is ready.

SINUSITIS

An inflamed sinus lining is known as sinusitis. Sinusitis is a viral infection, but other factors, like smoking, weak immunity, seasonal allergies, etc., can also trigger this infection. Fungal or bacterial sinusitis is very rare but exists. **The known symptoms of sinusitis are nasal discharge, inflammation in the sinuses, headache, and congestion.**

NATURAL REMEDIES

1. **Essential Oils:** You can inhale oils like tea tree and eucalyptus directly from the bottle by adding in a diffuser or through steam. Mix 100ml of fatty acid-containing oil with 2ml each of clove, lavender, pine, and thyme oil. Rub the mixture on the affected area or add a few drops in your nostrils.
2. **Vitamin C Diet:** Take vitamin-enriched food like cayenne, orange, garlic, etc., daily. Garlic also clears mucus congestion caused by sinusitis.
3. **Red Root:** Take 30–50 drops of red root tincture five times per week. Reduce the dose to half for kids.
4. **Saline Solution Rinse:** Make a 60% saline solution (mix 60g of salt in your desired volume of water) and rinse the nasal cavity a few times a day.
5. **Mucous Clearing Tea:** Taking 1-2 cups of this tea will clear out the mucous. Boil one tsp of willow bark and bayberry root in two cups of water until the water remains half. Stain the water and drink.

Recipe for Treating Sinusitis

Recipe: Sinus Tea

Ingredients:
- 1 cup of warm water
- 1 tsp of raw, unfiltered honey
- 1/2 lemon, juiced
- 1-2 slices of fresh ginger
- A pinch of cayenne pepper
- A pinch of salt

Instructions:
- Combine the warm water, honey, and lemon juice in a cup.
- Add the slices of fresh ginger.
- Add cayenne pepper to help with congestion and as an anti-inflammatory.
- If you're not on a sodium-restricted diet, add a little salt to help soothe your throat and thin mucus.
- Add honey for sweetness and dissolve properly.
- Drink the warm mixture gently to let the ingredients and steam help clear your sinuses and comfort your throat.

SNORING

The vibration of relaxed throat tissues during sleep produces a harsh sound called snoring. A few reasons for snoring are lack of sleep, wrong sleep position, blocked nasal passage, sedative medicines, or alcohol use. **The signs of snoring are high blood pressure, dry throat, headache, and choking at night.**

NATURAL REMEDIES

1. **Peppermint Oil:** Inhaling peppermint oil before bedtime may help clear nasal passages and reduce snoring. Add a few drops in a hot water bowl to take steam.
2. **Avoid Sedatives and Alcohol:** Alcohol and sedatives relax throat muscles, making snoring more likely. Avoid them, especially in the evening.
3. **Lose Weight and Stay Hydrated:** Losing excess weight will alleviate the pressure on your airways and decrease snoring. Staying well-hydrated can help prevent mucus from becoming sticky, which can contribute to snoring.
4. **Spearmint and Peppermint:** Chewing spearmint and peppermint can also reduce snoring. These herbs will clear the nasal passage because of their mentholated properties that reduce snoring.
5. **Fenugreek:** Soak a tsp of fenugreek seeds overnight, then drink the water in the morning to help alleviate nasal congestion and reduce snoring.
6. **Ginger Tea:** Ginger promotes saliva production that hydrates the throat and reduces snoring; take a cup of ginger tea before sleep.

SORE THROAT

Viral infections, allergens, and colds cause soreness in the upper respiratory tract. This condition irritates the throat and causes pain when swallowing. **A sore throat is characterized by inflamed lymph nodes, pain, fever, hoarse sound production, and scratchy throat.**

NATURAL REMEDIES

1. **Thyme:** Use this herb to make tea or gargle with thyme water for soothing properties.
2. **Saline Water Wash:** Make 60% salted water and gargle a few times daily for sore throat symptoms.
3. **Calendula:** Take a handful of dried flowers and steep in boiled water for 15 minutes. Strain and drink the water.
4. **Licorice Roots:** Chew fresh licorice or use dried roots to make tea.
5. **Andrographis:** You can take Andrographis supplements, extract, or make dried-leaf tea.
6. **Slippery Elm:** Chew the inner bark of slippery elm to soothe sore throat. Mucilage, a component of slippery elm, turns into a gel by mixing with water. This gel gives soothing effects for throat irritation.
7. **Honey:** Take a tbsp of honey to ease irritation and inflammation caused by sore throat.

Recipe: Herbal Tea

Ingredients:

- 1 tbsp of dried chamomile flowers
- 1 tbsp of dried peppermint leaves
- 1 tbsp of dried licorice root
- 2 cups of water
- Honey (optional, for sweetness)

Instructions:

- Boil water in a pot and add all the herbs in boiling water.
- Steep the herbs for 15 minutes on low flame until water remains half.
- Strain the tea and add honey (optional).
- Take 1-2 cups of this tea daily.

SPRAINS

A sprain is called the stretching or tearing of ligaments around a joint that often causes pain and swelling. Trauma, impact, movement in unnatural positions, and overstretching/tearing of ligaments due to sudden twisting can cause sprains. **The signs of sprains are inflammation, bruising, sharp pain, joint stiffness, and limited movement.**

NATURAL REMEDIES

1. **Alder:** You can use alder bark to make a tonic and apply it to the affected area.
2. **Comfrey:** Apply comfrey leaves poultice on effective areas to treat sprains.
3. **Arnica:** Use arnica flowers to make infused oil, tinctures, or paste and apply to the affected area.
4. **Epsom Salt:** Add 1-2 cups of salt in warm water and soak your body for 10-15 minutes in it. You can also mix a few drops of peppermint oil for better results.
5. **Turmeric:** Make turmeric paste in water and apply it to the affected area to ease symptoms of sprains.
6. **Peppermint Oil and Aloe Vera Gel:** Mix 8-10 drops of oil in 2 tbsp gel and apply on the affected area a few times daily.

<u>**Recipe for Treating Sprains**</u>

Recipe: Ginger-Comfrey Balm

Ingredients:

- 1/2 cup dried comfrey leaves
- 2 tbsp grated fresh ginger
- 1 cup carrier oil
- 2 tbsp beeswax
- 10-15 drops of lavender oil

Instructions:

- Add ginger, comfrey roots, and carrier oil to a cooker. Let the ingredients cook for 3-5 hours on low flame.
- Filter the oil with cheesecloth and remove ginger and comfrey. Let the oil cool down a bit.
- Melt beeswax in a double-boiler and mix with infused oil. Add lavender oil for aroma.
- Pour the mixture into a clean jar and let it cool and solidify.
- Apply the balm on the affected area and cover it with a cold pack for 15 minutes. Repeat the process a few times a day.

STOMACH FLU

Infection of the intestine and stomach is called stomach. It's also known as gastroenteritis. Although the virus is the primary cause of stomach flu, chemicals, parasites, and bacteria can also be the factors. **This infection is characterized by low fever, nausea, vomiting, abdominal pain, loss of appetite, stomach cramps and pain, and Diarrhea.**

NATURAL REMEDIES

1. **Prunella:** Use the leaves and stem of the plant in tea or salad to cure stomach flu.
2. **Musta:** Consume 1-2 tsp of dried musta roots in the form of tea.
3. **Bael/Bilva:** Prepare a mixture by mixing Bael pulp or juice with a little water. Consume this mixture to help soothe digestive discomfort, reduce Diarrhea, and alleviate stomach flu symptoms.
4. **Ginger:** You can make ginger tea by soaking fresh ginger roots in hot water. Drink slowly to soothe your stomach.
5. **Peppermint Oil:** Inhaling the aroma of peppermint oil or taking its capsules thrice daily will help deal with stomach flu.

Recipe for Treating Stomach Flu

Recipe: Stomach-Soothing Tea
Ingredients:

- 1 tsp dried chamomile flowers
- 1 tsp dried peppermint leaves
- 1 tsp dried ginger root slices
- 1 cup drinking water
- Honey

Instructions:

- Boil water in a kettle.
- Steep all the herbs in boiled water for 10-15 minutes.
- Strain the water and add honey (if sweetness is required)
- Drink the tea slowly for good results.

STRESS AND ANXIETY

Stress is a physiological response to external pressures or demands. Anxiety is a persistent feeling of unease or fear caused due to threats. Both of these conditions affect a person's physical and mental health. **The significant signs of stress and anxiety are sleeplessness, stomachache, high blood pressure, headache, weight loss, dizziness, and difficulty breathing.**

NATURAL REMEDIES

1. **Deep Breathing:** Practice deep breathing exercises to relax your nervous system. Inhale deeply through your nose, hold for four seconds, and exhale. Repeat several times.
2. **Meditation:** Regular meditation can reduce stress and anxiety. Use guided meditation apps to help you get started.
3. **Aromatherapy:** Sniffing the aroma of any essential oil, like neroli, lavender, jasmine, Bergamot, chamomile, etc., will give you calming effects.
4. **Chamomile Tea:** Thai tea is a natural sedative that can help reduce anxiety and promote better sleep.
5. **Lemon Balm:** Lemon balm has strong anti-anxiety properties that last for about 4 hours. You can consume it in the form of herbal tea or capsules. Lemon balm combination with other herbs like valerian will increase its effects.
6. **Alfalfa:** Add the sprouts raw or leaves of this plant to your diet. You can also use ashwagandha as an alfalfa alternative.

Recipe for Treating Stress and Anxiety

Recipe: Stress-Reducing Smoothie

Ingredients:
- 1 medium banana
- 1/2 cup Greek yogurt
- 1/2 cup blueberries
- 1 tbsp honey
- 1/2 tsp ground cinnamon
- 1/2 tsp powdered ashwagandha
- 1/2 cup unsweetened almond milk
- Ice cubes (optional)

Instructions:
- Add everything in a blender and blend them until a smooth texture is obtained.
- Maintain the consistency and sweetness of the smoothie according to desire.
- Add ice cubes and mix again.
- Take one glass of this fresh smoothie every day.

STUFFY NOSE

The inflamed tissue wall inside the nose causes a congested or stuffy nose. Factors like cold, allergen, infection, or inflamed blood vessels can cause a stuffy nose. **This condition is characterized by fullness or blockage of the nasal cavity, pain, breathing difficulty, headache, lethargy, cough, and sneezing.**

NATURAL REMEDIES

1. **Peppermint:** You can use peppermint in different ways, like sniffing peppermint oil, adding oil to water to wash your face, or having a cup of peppermint leaves tea.
2. **Rosemary:** Inhale rosemary oil directly from a bottle or through steam, or massage it on your nostrils with olive oil.
3. **Green Tea:** Green tea treats stuffy nose, clears respiratory tract infections, and eases sore throat. Have 1-2 cups of tea daily.
4. **Honey and Lemon:** Mix one tsp of lemon juice in one tsp of honey and drink twice daily. You can add them to any herbal tea as well.
5. **Ginger Tea:** Make ginger tea or add fresh ginger to your green tea.

Recipe for Treating Stuffy Nose

Recipe: Homemade Vapor Rub

Ingredients:
- 1/2 cup coconut oil
- 2 tbsp beeswax pellets
- 20 drops of eucalyptus oil
- 10 drops of peppermint oil
- 10 drops of lavender oil (optional)

Instructions:
- Melt and mix the coconut oil and beeswax in a double boiler.
- After the mixture cools slightly, add the above essential oils and mix well. Lavender oil is optional.
- Pour the mixture into a jar and let it solidify.
- Gently rub this gel on your nostrils, throat, chest, and back.
- The soothing blend will help relieve congestion and promote easier breathing.

SUNBURN

Sunburn is caused by prolonged skin exposure to UV light from the sun or any other source. **This condition results in redness, blisters, chills, burning, swollen, and dry skin.** Sunburn is prevalent in sensitive and light skin tones with low melanin production. Melanin is a compound naturally produced by the skin that blocks UV rays.

NATURAL REMEDIES

1. **Rosemary, Carrot, and Aloe Gel:** Rosemary oil contains cooling properties that reduce sunburn irritations. Carrot seed oil promotes healing, while aloe vera gel has anti-inflammatory properties and keeps the burned skin hydrated and smooth. Mix 20 drops each of rosemary and carrot oil with a cup of aloe gel and pour in a spray bottle. Spray the affected area a few times a day.
2. **Sesame and Sea Buckthorn Oil Solution:** Combining sesame and sea buckthorn oil will treat sunburns and replenish your skin. Mix one tbsp of buckthorn oil with 7 tbsp of sesame oil and apply on your skin twice a day.
3. **Witch Hazel:** Apply witch hazel oil or extract on burned skin or mix with aloe gel.
4. **Hyssop-Aloe Combination:** Make hyssop infusion by adding 2 tbsp in half a cup of water. Strain the water, mix with ¼ cup of aloe gel, and apply burns.
5. **Oatmeal Bath:** Tie the oatmeal on the faucet opening with cheesecloth or sock and fill the tub. Take a bath with oatmeal water.
6. **Tea Bags:** Apply cooled water-soaked tea bags on sunburned skin to relieve pain and swelling.
7. **Coconut Oil:** Applying coconut oil on sunburned skin will prevent the condition from worsening and promote healing.

Recipe for Treating Sunburn

Recipe: Calendula Healing Salve

Ingredients:
- 1 cup dried calendula flowers
- 16 ounces avocado oil/extra-virgin olive oil
- 4 ounces beeswax pellets.

Instructions:
- Add dried leaves and oil in a double boiler and cook on low flame until the leaves turn light brown or yellow.
- Strain the oil from the leaves with cheesecloth.
- Melt the beeswax in another double boiler. Let the wax cool down a bit.
- Add calendula-infused oil to melted beeswax and mix.
- Pour the paste into a clean jar and let it solidify. You can store it for a year.
- Use this salve directly on the sunburn area a few times a day.

SWEATING AND BODY ODOR

Sweating and body odor are natural processes. Between 2 different sweat glands, "apocrine" is the one that produces body odor. These mechanisms are natural but can be unpleasant and promote bacterial growth on the skin. However, there are many ways to reduce sweat and odor production from the body.

NATURAL REMEDIES

1. **Essential Oils:** Apply a few drops of available oil (Patchouli, Neroli, lavender, Tea tree, Eucalyptus, or Bergamot) to your body after the bath. These oils also have fungal and bacterial killing properties that cause body odor after sweating.
2. **Apple Cider Vinegar:** Apply apple cider vinegar to the excessive sweating areas to prevent odor. To use the vinegar, dilute it with water in equal parts and apply to clean, dry skin. Let it air dry before dressing to balance pH levels and control odor.

Note: Perform a patch test first to ensure it doesn't irritate your skin.

3. **Sage:** Use 3 tsp of dried leaves to make sage tea and drink 3 times daily.
4. **Camphor:** Apply a few drops of Camphor oil as a natural deodorant and antibacterial agent.
5. **Cornstarch and Baking Soda:** Mix cornstarch and baking soda equally and apply on your feet and underarms to prevent excessive sweating and oil production. Add essential oil for aroma.
6. **Hydro Solution:** Mix one tsp of hydrogen peroxide in a cup of water and apply it to the sweat area to reduce bacterial production.
7. **Aloe Zest:** Mix 6 drops each of lavender and eucalyptus oil in ¼ cup of aloe gel and spray on the excessive sweating area. The essential oils will provide aroma and are bactericidal, while the aloe gel has antibacterial properties.

Recipe for Treating Sweating and Body Odor

Recipe: Natural Deodorant

Ingredients:

- 3 tbsp of coconut oil
- 2 tbsp cocoa butter
- 2 tbsp of shea butter
- 2 tbsp of beeswax pellets
- 2 tbsp of baking soda
- 2 tbsp of arrowroot powder/cornstarch
- 8 drops of essential oils

Instructions:

- Melt coconut butter, shea butter, and beeswax in a double boiler.
- After everything melts, add coconut oil, essential oil of your choice, baking soda, and arrowroot powder to the mixture and mix well.
- Let the mixture cool slightly and pour in a clean jar.
- Apply on areas with excessive sweat production.

TENDER BREASTS

Breasts that are sensitive, stiff, sore, or painful to touch are called tender breasts. It happens due to hormonal changes like pregnancy or menstrual, child feeding, and adolescence. **The common symptoms are swelling, sharp stabbing pain, and fullness or tightness of the breast.**

NATURAL REMEDIES

1. **Sweet Violet:** The massage of sweet violet oil once daily eases breast swelling and tenderness and softens lumps. Make the sweet violet-infused oil with 2.5 cups violet flowers and leaves in 3 cups almond oil.
2. **Ginkgo:** Gingko eases breast tenderness associated with the menstrual cycle. Consume 60-240 mg dosage of ginkgo in the form of leaf extract.

Note: Avoid using ginkgo during pregnancy because it can cause excessive bleeding during labor.

3. **Vitamin B6:** Vitamin B6 is effective in dealing with PMS symptoms like breast tenderness. It's recommended to consult a specialist before taking Vitamin B6.

Note: Only take 100mg/day as the high dose can be harmful.

4. **Warm Water Bath:** Mix 10 drops of lavender oil and two cups of Epsom salt in the bathtub and mix well in warm water. Soak your body in water for 10-15 minutes and relax.
5. **Nipple Soothing Cream:** Mix 55 g each of melted cocoa and shea butter in 281 g coconut oil. Apply the cream a few times daily to avoid nipple cracks caused by breastfeeding.

Recipe for Treating Tender Breast

Recipe: Flaxseeds and Raisin Muffins

Ingredients:

- 1 cup whole wheat flour
- 1/2 cup ground flaxseed
- 1/2 cup raisins
- 1/4 cup honey
- 1/4 cup unsweetened applesauce
- 1/4 cup plain yogurt
- 1/4 cup almond milk
- 2 eggs
- 2 tsp baking powder
- 1/2 tsp baking soda
- 1/2 tsp vanilla extract
- 1/2 tsp ground cinnamon
- 1/4 tsp salt

Instructions:

- Preheat the oven to 175°C.
- Mix all the powdered ingredients in a large bowl.
- Whisk the liquid ingredients in another bowl.
- Mix the wet and dry ingredients until combined.
- Gently fold the raisins into the muffin batter.
- Fill the muffin cups 2/3 with batter.
- Bake the muffins in the oven for 18-20 minutes until fully cooked.
- Allow the muffins to cool and serve.

TENDINITIS

An alignment caused by irritation or swelling of the tendon is tendinitis. The tendon is a thick cord that attaches muscles to bones. **Tendinitis is characterized by limited mobility, swelling, and pain that gets worse with overuse.** This condition can be caused by heavy exercise, overuse, injury or accident, disease, and aging.

NATURAL REMEDIES

1. **Arnica and Meadowsweet:** Make the herbal infused oil of one cup each of arnica and meadowsweet leaves and flowers in 3 cups of olive base oil. Mix the oil with 4 tbsp beeswax pellets for thickness. Massage this salve on the affected area 3 times daily.

2. **Solomon's Seal:** You can use the herbal roots of the Solomon seal to make tea. Place 1 Solomon's Seal Tea bag in a cup and add 100mL of hot water to get the maximum flavor out of each cup. Brew your tea for two to three minutes, then enjoy it!

3. **Turmeric-Ginger Tea:** Boil one tsp of turmeric powder and one tbsp of chopped ginger in a cup of water. Drink this tea 3 times daily.

4. **Peppermint Salve:** Add two oz of dried peppermint in a cup of extra-virgin olive oil to make peppermint-infused oil. Mix the infused oil with one oz of melted beeswax. Apply the salve on the affected tendons every 3 hours.

5. **Essential Oils:** Mix 2 tbsp of vegetable oil with 10 drops of essential oil and gently rub the affected area to relieve pain and inflammation.

6. **Dandelion Flower Oil:** Massage a few drops of this oil to reduce muscle soreness and joint pain.

Recipe for Treating Tendonitis

Recipe: Tendonitis Relief Balm
Ingredients:
- 1/2 cup coconut oil
- 2 tbsp grated beeswax
- 10-15 drops of essential oil
- 1-2 tsp of turmeric powder

Instructions:
- Melt the coconut oil and beeswax completely in the microwave until fully liquified.
- Allow the mixture to cool slightly.
- Stir in your chosen essential oil for fragrance and added soothing benefits.
- Mix turmeric powder into the mixture.
- Pour the balm into a clean container and let it solidify.
- Apply the balm on the inflamed tendon a few times a day.

TOOTHACHES

Toothaches are sharp or throbbing pain in and around a tooth or the jaw. Common symptoms include:

- Intense pain
- Hot or cold temperature sensitivity
- Swelling
- A foul taste in the mouth

This condition is caused due to tooth decay, gum disease, dental abscesses, cracked teeth, and sinus infections.

NATURAL REMEDIES

1. **Licorice:** Chew licorice roots to relieve toothache, soreness, sensitivity, and teeth cleaning.
2. **Tea Tree Mouth Rinse:** Rinse your mouth with the tea tree oil or mix the oil with vodka for numbing effects.
3. **Clove Oil and Salt:** Add three drops of clove oil and ¼ tsp of salt in a glass of warm water and rinse your mouth. This mouthwash will provide you with instant pain relief.
4. **Peppermint Tea:** Peppermint has numbing properties and can provide temporary relief from pain. Drink a cup of tea slowly to relieve pain.

Recipe for Treating Toothache

Recipe: Chamomile and Peppermint Tea

Ingredients:

- 1 chamomile tea bag
- 1 teaspoon of dried peppermint leaves
- 1 cup of boiling water
- Honey (optional, for sweetness)

Instructions:

- Put the dried peppermint leaves and chamomile tea bag in a cup.
- Cover the herbs with boiling water.
- Allow it to steep for five to ten minutes.
- Take out the tea bag, then remove the peppermint leaves.
- If you would like sweetness, add honey.
- Swirl the tea around on your lips before taking a calm, leisurely sip.

ULCER

Ulcers are lesions on the stomach or small intestine lining. Sores on your esophagus (throat) are another possibility. Gastric ulcers are stomach ulcers. Ulcer pain is a burning sensation inside the stomach. **Burning stomach pain, bloating, heartburn, loss of appetite, and nausea are the most obvious symptoms seen in ulcer patients.**

NATURAL REMEDIES

1. **Pineapple Weed:** Pineapple weed makes a delicious cup of tea. Fill a teapot with the necessary number of pineapple weed heads. Pour boiling water over the top and let steep for five minutes. Add sugar or honey (as needed).

2. **Baking Soda Mouth Paste:** Make a soothing mouth rinse by dissolving one or two tablespoons of baking soda in a glass of water. Apply it on the ulcer location to relieve pain. Repeat it as often as needed.

3. **Ginger:** You can add one tablespoon of fresh chopped ginger to 1 cup of boiling water to make ginger tea.

4. **Calendula Tea:** It is taken by mixing calendula leaves in hot water. It can soothe the discomfort of the throat and stomach ulcers.

5. **Onion:** You can add sliced onions to salads and sandwiches, stir-fries, fajitas, and pasta dishes.

Note: Be careful not to fry them, as this can irritate your stomach.

Recipe for Treating Ulcer

Recipe: Cabbage Juice Relief

Ingredients:
- ½ head white cabbage
- Washed and chopped coarsely (no hearts)
- About 2 cups (475 ml) water

Instructions:
- Fill a mixer halfway with cabbage.
- Fill the rest with water.
- The mixture should be strained or pressed. (To strain out the juice, use a medium-sized French press.) Twelve cups (120 ml) can be consumed up to three times daily.
- Keep any leftovers in the refrigerator. After twenty-four hours, discard.

URINARY TRACT INFECTIONS

UTIs are frequent illnesses when bacteria enter the urethra and infect the urinary system, usually through the skin or rectum. The parts of the urinary system include the kidney, ureter, bladder, and urethra. **Pelvic pain, a burning sensation when peeing, frequent urination, dark urine, and strong odor of urine are the most prominent symptoms of UTI.**

NATURAL REMEDIES

1. **Angelica:** One teaspoon of dried angelica root should be added to a glass of boiling water, covered, and allowed to steep for 10 to 15 minutes. Drink once or twice daily.

2. **Berry Juice:** Mix 1 cup of berries and with ¾ cup rice milk in a blender to make it smooth. Add ¾ cups of ice to it and drink once or twice daily. You can use bearberry, raspberry, or cranberry to treat UTIs.

3. **Urva Ursi:** One dose is made using 2 teaspoons of dried urva ursi leaves or 4 teaspoons of fresh urva ursi leaves and 2 cups of water.

4. **Supplements of Garlic:** You can take 9 cloves of raw garlic daily and divide it into 3 doses to treat urinary tract infections.

5. **Baking Soda:** It is suggested that you mix 1/2 to 1 teaspoon of baking soda with water and drink it first thing in the morning. It can help with this illness.

Precaution: Once you've eliminated the illness, cease taking it.

Recipe for Treating UTI

Recipe: Cranberry Juice
Ingredients:
- 2 quarter water
- Honey to taste
- 8 cups fresh cranberries
- ½ cup lemon juice
- ½ cup orange juice

Instructions:
- Put water and cranberries in a large saucepan to boil for 5 minutes.
- Lower the heat and cover the pan. Leave the mixture for 25 minutes.
- Add lemon juice and orange juice. Mix it and add honey to taste.
- Allow it to cool down before serving.
- Add ice to enjoy it.

VAGINAL DISCHARGE

Vaginal discharge is a clear, white, or off-white fluid that leaks from your cervix. The signs of vaginal infection are **thick white discharge, bad odor, pain in the lower abdomen, and bumps in the genital area.**

NATURAL REMEDIES

1. **Geranium:** Mix 1 ounce of warm spring water with 3 ounces of yogurt. Add three drops of geranium. Twice daily, irrigate your vagina with the yogurt mixture after placing it in a douche.

2. **Greek Yogurt:** When treating a yeast infection with yogurt, choose plain Greek yogurt. Make sure the yogurt has no added sugar, flavoring, or fruit. Remove a tampon from the applicator. Yogurt should be inserted into your vagina using the applicator after being filled with yogurt. Alternatively, you can insert as much as possible with your fingers into your vagina.

3. **Essential Oil of Oregano:** Take 3-5 drops/ounce of oil in a jar. The oil can be almond oil, olive oil, or any other. Add crushed oregano leaves. Place the jar in a saucepan of hot water for 15 minutes. Place the jar in a sunny window for 1-2 weeks. Massage it onto your skin or inhale it through a diffuser.
4. **Coconut Oil:** You can use coconut oil by putting on a fresh tampon before inserting it to treat vaginal infections.
5. **Apple Cider Vinegar:** Adding a half cup of apple cider vinegar to a lukewarm bathtub and soaking your body for 20 minutes may help eradicate hazardous germs, including yeast.
6. **Hydrogen Peroxide:** Antiseptic hydrogen peroxide can kill germs and yeast. Lactobacillus bacteria in your vagina produce hydrogen peroxide as part of their natural biological activity. It may assist with yeast growth on the genitals if you add it to a bath or dilute it in water before applying it to your skin. Dilute by adding equal parts of water and hydrogen peroxide.

VARICOSE VEINS

The term "varicose" is derived from the Latin word "varix," which means "twisted." Varicose veins are bluish-purple, twisted veins that are swollen and twisted. Because leg veins must fight against gravity, varicose veins are most common on the legs. **Aching, heavy, and unpleasant legs are among the major symptoms.**

NATURAL REMEDIES

1. **Horse Chestnut:** You can apply horse chestnut oil directly to the legs to treat this illness.
2. **Plant Extract with Essential Oils:** Dilute plant extracts and essential oils in carrier oils before applying topically or using an aromatherapy diffuser.
3. **Flavonoids:** Leafy vegetables, onion, spinach, apple, cherries, berries, and citrus fruits such as lemon, orange, and grapefruit are major sources of flavonoids. You can eat vegetables in cooked form and take the juices of fruits to treat varicose veins.
4. **Witch Hazel:** Apply a witch hazel-dipped washcloth to the affected region. Try to do this twice or thrice daily for a month or two. Alternately, add 10 to 20 drops of distilled witch hazel to a tub of warm water. Spend at least 15 minutes soaking your legs in the solution.
5. **Butcher's Broom:** The root of the butcher's broom is crushed and made into powder form. You can take 1.5-3 grams per day to treat varicose veins.

Recipe for Treating Varicose Veins

Recipe: Calendula Vein Liniment
Ingredients:
- 2 tablespoons dried calendula
- 2 tablespoons yarrow
- 1 tablespoon self-heal herb
- Approx. 100 ml distilled witch hazel water

Instructions:

- Pour enough witch hazel to cover the dry herbs and leave to macerate for 2 weeks.
- Bottle after straining and store in the refrigerator.
- Apply topically to inflamed regions and varicose veins. The simplest method is to dampen muslin and cut a piece large enough to cover the named area.

WARTS

A verruca is a scientific term for a wart, tiny skin growth caused by any of 60 related human papillomavirus strains that affect the skin's surface layer or epidermis. **A small bump on the skin that can range from 1-10mm, rough or smooth surface, may be in clusters, and itching are the signs of warts.** Face, feet, and knees are mostly affected with this ailment.

NATURAL REMEDIES

1. **Basil:** If you'd prefer not to use fresh basil, you can substitute a drop or two of its essential oil for this treatment. You can apply basil oil directly to the skin twice daily.
2. **Garlic Oil:** This cure requires more preparation time than a fresh garlic compress, but it saves you time and effort in the long run. If you also apply raw honey to the treated wart, with antiviral characteristics, your wart may go even faster. You have to peel out the garlic and heat it in any essential oil, such as olive oil, for 20 minutes to make garlic oil. Do not overheat.
3. **Fresh Celandine:** Break off a fresh plant leaf or stem and apply the latex (plant fluid; in this example, orange-yellow) directly to the wart's center. Do this twice a day for two weeks.
4. **Lemon Balm:** Extracts of this minty, lemony herb are extremely antiviral. Placing a leaf over the wart or applying tincture/essential oil directly on warts over time may hasten removal and shrinking.
5. **Dandelions:** Break apart a dandelion and squeeze out the sticky white fluid to try this procedure. Apply once or twice a day on the wart. Repeat for another two weeks.
6. **Castor Oil:** Apply castor oil to the wart daily. The wart may fall off after two or more weeks.

WRINKLES

Wrinkles, a common indicator of aging, are significantly easier to prevent than remove. Herbs, like cosmetics, will not suddenly eliminate your crow's feet and fine wrinkles; they may help you obtain smoother-looking skin organically. The symptoms of aging or wrinkles are **creases or folds on the skin, fine lines around the lips and eyes, and loose skin.**

NATURAL REMEDIES

1. **Pomegranate Oil:** Buy pomegranate oil from any store. Apply this oil to wrinkles by gently massaging a few drops onto clean and dry skin before bedtime.
2. **Rosehip Seed Oil:** You can prepare the oil at home by soaking a cup of dried rosehip seeds in a jar full of carrier oil. Place the pot for 3 weeks in a dark place. Stain the oil and use it.

3. **Aloe Vera:** To use Aloe Vera for wrinkles, apply pure Aloe Vera gel to clean the skin, massage it in gently, and leave it on without rinsing. Use it daily for potential skin hydration and collagen production benefits to help reduce the appearance of wrinkles over time.

4. **Witch Hazel:** Apply pure witch hazel extract to clean skin using a cotton ball. Allow it to dry and moisturize afterward. Use it twice daily, but start slowly to check any skin's reaction.

5. **Egg White:** To use egg white for wrinkle treatment, whisk it, apply it to your clean face, let it dry for 15-20 minutes, and then rinse off with lukewarm water. It can temporarily tighten the skin and reduce the appearance of wrinkles when used 1-2 times a week.

6. **Yogurt Mask:** Mix 1 tbsp of plain yogurt with a tsp of honey and a few drops of lemon juice. Apply this mixture to your face and neck for 15-20 minutes, then rinse with warm water. Use this mask 1-2 times a week for smoother, more youthful-looking skin.

7. **Coconut Oil:** Gently massage a small amount of coconut oil onto clean skin in upward, circular motions, focusing on wrinkle-prone areas. Use it consistently until wrinkles disappear.

- X -

Hello,

Thank you for reading one of my books. As an alternative medicine practitioner, I tried to compile 500+ natural remedies and 100+ recipes for 110 most common ailments and everyday illnesses. If you have really enjoyed this book and found it useful, please take a few moments to write a <u>review</u> of it. Please scan the following code to review this book. Thank you!

PAUL DEV

www.ingramcontent.com/pod-product-compliance
Lightning Source LLC
Chambersburg PA
CBHW080850260726
48660CB00009B/3259